Preventing Hospital Infections

Preventing Hospital Infections

Real-World Problems, Realistic Solutions

SECOND EDITION

JENNIFER MEDDINGS

VINEET CHOPRA

AND

SANJAY SAINT

OXFORD
UNIVERSITY PRESS

OXFORD
UNIVERSITY PRESS

Oxford University Press is a department of the University of Oxford. It furthers the University's objective of excellence in research, scholarship, and education by publishing worldwide. Oxford is a registered trade mark of Oxford University Press in the UK and certain other countries.

Published in the United States of America by Oxford University Press
198 Madison Avenue, New York, NY 10016, United States of America.

First Edition published in 2015
Second Edition published in 2021

Library of Congress Cataloging-in-Publication Data
Names: Meddings, Jennifer author. | Chopra, Vineet author. | Saint, Sanjay author.
Title: Preventing hospital infections : real-world problems, realistic solutions /
Jennifer Meddings, Vineet Chopra, Sanjay Saint.
Description: Second edition. | New York, NY : Oxford University Press, [2021] |
Preceded by Preventing hospital infections / Sanjay Saint, Sarah L. Krein. 2015. |
Includes bibliographical references and index.
Identifiers: LCCN 2020047013 (print) | LCCN 2020047014 (ebook) |
ISBN 9780197509159 (paperback) | ISBN 9780197509173 (epub) | ISBN 9780197509180
Subjects: MESH: Cross Infection—prevention & control | Catheter-Related
Infections—prevention & control | Clostridium Infections—prevention & control |
Equipment Contamination—prevention & control | Infectious Disease Transmission,
Professional-to-Patient—prevention & control | Infection Control Practitioners |
Guideline Adherence
Classification: LCC RC683.5.I5 (print) | LCC RC683.5.I5 (ebook) |
NLM WX 167 | DDC 617/.05—dc23
LC record available at https://lccn.loc.gov/2020047013
LC ebook record available at https://lccn.loc.gov/2020047014

DOI: 10.1093/med/9780197509159.001.0001

9 8 7 6 5 4 3 2 1

Printed by Marquis, Canada

To my parents, Betty and Leo Meddings, for their endless support, and to my patients and their families for the privilege of caring for them.
Jennifer Meddings

To Palak, Vyaan, and Priya. Thank you for making me complete.
Vineet Chopra

To my nursing colleagues throughout the world: Thank you for your tireless efforts in caring for patients.
Sanjay Saint

CONTENTS

Nearly 2 million Americans develop a healthcare-associated infection each year, and some 100,000 of them die as a result. Yet healthcare-associated infections are reasonably preventable through hospitals' adoption and implementation of evidence-based methods that offer sizable potential savings—in terms of both lives and dollars. A major stumbling block exists between these preventive methods and their full implementation, namely, the failure of large numbers of healthcare personnel to put the methods into practice.

First, though, we would like to pause a moment to acknowledge the altered healthcare environment into which this book is being launched. We had no idea when we set forth on the new edition that it would appear while the world was still reeling from the effects of a very different kind of infection. Our hearts go out to those whose lives have been torn apart by the novel coronavirus pandemic.

There is no shortage of books that address healthcare-associated infection and its prevention. Most of them, however, are primarily focused on identifying and describing the various types of infection and on the "technical" aspects of prevention—the sanitary conditions or the latest device that will stop germs from spreading. The "adaptive aspects"—the acceptance and use of preventive measures by clinical personnel—receive relatively little attention.

This book, now in its second edition, is primarily devoted to that very issue, providing detailed guidance for dealing with the human equation in a hospital quality improvement initiative. We address that challenge in every element of an initiative, from the decision by senior leaders to proceed, to the selection of a project manager and physician and nurse champions, to the piloting of the initiative on a single medical unit and its rollout to the entire hospital or system, to the sustaining of the project's gains. There are chapters that pinpoint the main categories of resistance to an initiative and how to cope with them, that analyze the role of leadership in a change initiative, and that explore the future of infection prevention. All of the chapters have been carefully updated since the first edition, with new (or expanded) material on the technical aspects of preventing several types of hospital infection; tools and algorithms that can be used by front-line providers as well as more senior managers; appropriateness criteria for using invasive urinary and vascular access devices; recent results of several large collaborative infection prevention studies; novel approaches, including mindfulness and motivational interviewing to change behavior; and the role of the patient and family in preventing infection. We have been greatly appreciative of the positive feedback we received on the first edition; we hope this latest iteration continues to meet the needs of our readers. In order to provide a fresh perspective, we have added two new authors, each with deep expertise in this topic. We are also extremely grateful to Dr. Sarah Krein for her work on the first edition; much of the material in this book reflects her important contributions.

The book follows an infection prevention initiative as it might unfold in a model hospital. Because the initiative we use addresses catheter-associated urinary tract infection (CAUTI), it involves the entire hospital and the whole range of clinical staff, rather than being limited to, say, the emergency department or the intensive care unit. As a result, we believe its lessons can be applied to many other kinds of quality improvement efforts, such as those to prevent venous thromboembolism and falls.

The book is relatively concise and written in a conversational style. Its content largely reflects our findings and the work that we have been engaged in over the last two decades in trying to understand why some hospitals are more successful than others in preventing healthcare-associated infection. This includes research and prevention-related activities funded by the Department of Veterans Affairs (VA), the National Institutes of Health (NIH), the Agency for Healthcare Research and Quality (AHRQ), the Centers for Disease Control and Prevention (CDC), the Health Research & Educational Trust (HRET) of the American Hospital Association, the Blue Cross Blue Shield of Michigan Foundation, and the Michigan Health and Hospital Association's Keystone Center.

In addition to the valuable support of our funders, we have been fortunate to work with a superb group of individuals who share our goal of preventing infection and enhancing patient safety. We are ever grateful to our dedicated project staff, including Karen Fowler, Jessica Ameling, Latoya Kuhn, Martha Quinn, Molly Harrod, Debbie Zawol, David Ratz, Michele Mazlin, and Rachel Ehrlinger. We have benefited greatly from our fruitful collaborations with a large number of individuals from different parts of the world, including Sarah Krein, Molly Harrod, Jane Forman, Valerie Vaughn, Tim Hofer, Mohamad Fakih, Russ Olmsted, Milisa Manojlovich, Lona Mody, Todd Greene, Sam Watson, Scott Flanders, Hugo Sax, Benedetta Allegranzi, Alessandro Bartoloni, Akihiko Saitoh, Anita Huis, Didier Pittet, Laraine Washer, Anucha Apisarnthanarak, Bob Wachter, Jay Bhatt, and Yasuharu Tokuda. We are especially grateful for the contributions to this work provided by Robert Stock—his quick eye and even quicker pen are greatly appreciated.

We also value the support we have received from our employers: the VA Ann Arbor Healthcare System and the University of Michigan. Both organizations are committed to excellence in all that they do, and we are honored to call both organizations our home. We remain grateful to our many supervisors through the years who have provided us with the support and encouragement to conduct our work, including Rod Hayward, Larry McMahon, John Carethers, Mark Hausman, Eve Kerr, Eric Young, Ginny Creasman, and Robert McDivitt. We also thank the many healthcare providers and administrators who participated in our interviews and shared with us their stories (trials, tribulations, and successes) as they worked to prevent infections in their organizations. It is these individuals and their counterparts in hospitals across the United States and the world for whom this book is primarily intended as we collectively strive to improve the safety of hospitalized patients.

Let the journey continue!

Jennifer Meddings
Vineet Chopra
Sanjay Saint

Jennifer Meddings, MD, MSc, is an associate professor of internal medicine and pediatrics at the University of Michigan Health System and the VA Ann Arbor Healthcare System. Much of her recent research has focused on evaluation and development of evidence-based interventions for prevention of catheter-associated urinary tract infection (CAUTI). She has performed several systematic reviews involving interventions to reduce unnecessary catheter use, including meta-analyses demonstrating that the use of urinary catheter reminders and stop orders can reduce CAUTIs by over 50%. Her work has informed the development and evaluation of educational interventions in multiple national collaboratives to reduce CAUTI in the acute care and long-term care settings. She developed and led a project using the RAND/UCLA Appropriateness Method to formally rate the appropriateness of three types of urinary catheters (indwelling, intermittent straight, and external) for hundreds of clinical scenarios commonly encountered in hospitalized adults on medical services; this work was published in *Annals of Internal Medicine*. She also applied the RAND/UCLA Appropriateness Method to generate the Michigan Appropriate Perioperative Criteria for common procedures in general surgery and orthopedics, published in *BMJ Quality & Safety*. Her work has also focused on the evaluation of measures of urinary catheter use for surveillance and public reporting and the challenges in implementing value-based purchasing programs that use metrics involving urinary catheter use and pressure ulcer development. She received her Medical

Doctorate from the University of Michigan, completed a medical residency and chief residency at the Ohio State University, and obtained a Master of Science in Health and Healthcare Research from the University of Michigan.

Vineet Chopra, MD, MSc, is chief of the Division of Hospital Medicine, associate professor of internal medicine at the University of Michigan, and a research scientist at the VA Ann Arbor Healthcare System. Dr. Chopra is an internationally recognized expert in patient safety. His research on the appropriateness of vascular access device use and its outcomes has informed clinical policies and protocols for countless hospitals and health systems. He is the recipient of numerous teaching and research awards, including the 2016 Kaiser Permanente Award for Clinical Teaching and the 2019 Distinguished Mentor Award from the Michigan Institute for Clinical and Health Research. Dr. Chopra has published over 200 peer-reviewed articles in journals such as *JAMA*, *Annals of Internal Medicine*, *BMJ*, *Lancet*, *Infection Control and Hospital Epidemiology*, and *Clinical Infectious Diseases*; the majority of these articles focused on preventing infectious and noninfectious complications from the use of vascular access devices.

Sanjay Saint, MD, MPH, MACP, is the chief of medicine at the VA Ann Arbor Healthcare System, the George Dock Professor of internal medicine at the University of Michigan, and the director of the VA/University of Michigan Patient Safety Enhancement Program. His research focuses on enhancing patient safety by preventing hospital infection and translating research findings into practice. He has authored over 375 peer-reviewed papers, approximately 110 of which appeared in the *New England Journal of Medicine*, *JAMA*, *Lancet*, or the *Annals of Internal Medicine*. He is an international leader in preventing CAUTI. He is a special correspondent to the *New England Journal of Medicine*, an editorial board member of *BMJ Quality and Safety*, an elected member of the American Society for Clinical Investigation and the Association of American Physicians, and an international honorary fellow of the Royal College of Physicians

(FRCP). He received his Medical Doctorate from UCLA, completed a medical residency and chief residency at the University of California at San Francisco, and obtained a master's in public health (as a Robert Wood Johnson Clinical Scholar) from the University of Washington in Seattle. He has been a visiting professor at over 100 universities and hospitals in the United States, Europe, and Asia.

Preventing Hospital Infections

1

An Effective Strategy to Combat
Hospital Infections

The hospital is altogether the most complex human organization ever devised.

—Peter Drucker

We were interviewing staff members at a dozen hospitals that had taken part in a campaign to reduce healthcare-associated urinary tract infections. The goal was to make sure that indwelling urinary catheters were only used when medically necessary and were removed promptly when no longer needed, which sounded simple enough. But, in reality, it turned out to be infinitely complex and confusing.

We discovered, for example, that there were two sets of nurses who were worried about their patients taking a fall. One set wanted the catheter out as soon as possible because it interfered with patient mobility, and they feared that their patients, especially those who are a bit confused and do not even realize the catheter is in place, might trip on the tubing. "They are going to try and get out of bed and injure themselves," one nurse said.

Another set of nurses favored maintaining the catheter in place as long as possible because it tended to keep their patients in bed. A nurse put it this way, "Well, do I really want this person hopping out of bed, and can

I really be sure that they're going to call me to help them? We don't want there to be any falls."

Two groups of nurses that were both concerned about their patients' well-being; one group gladly cooperated with an infection prevention program, while the other group was, at best, reluctant. As is so often true when a hospital embarks on a campaign to control infection, the human dimension intruded.

There is universal agreement within the nation's hospitals that the prevention of healthcare-associated infection (HAI) is an absolute necessity for both humane and financial reasons. And there is no shortage of evidence-based strategies that can take us closer to that goal. Multiple studies[1-6] have demonstrated that at least 20% of all HAIs can be prevented, and some researchers have suggested that the figure might reach 70%; preventability appears to vary by the type of HAI and the clinical setting (within or outside an intensive care unit [ICU], for example). Yet many of the efforts that hospitals have made to implement these proven strategies have fallen short of their goals. Why? Our research spanning two decades has shown that a principal reason is the failure of the hospitals to win their staff's active support of infection prevention initiatives. In their focus on the technical aspects of an initiative, some hospitals have given short shrift to the human aspects imperative for improving patient safety.

We offer a field-tested framework for organizing and implementing a hospital-based initiative to combat infection. It includes descriptions and explanations of some evidence-based infection prevention procedures, but the major focus is on ways to inspire full-scale adoption of these practices—essentially, to change behavior. We answer this central question: Given all the complexities of the hospital operation—the hierarchical arrangements, the competing priorities, the web of personal relationships—how do you get the people of a hospital to truly buy in to an infection prevention initiative?

The stakes are high, and they can be quickly stated. A multistate point prevalence study published in 2018 estimated that in 2015 there were 687,200 hospital-acquired infections in US hospitals.[3] The infections create physical and emotional distress for hundreds of thousands of patients annually. They also take a psychological toll on the staff of a hospital and on its culture, constant reminders of their failure to live up to their credo, *primum non nocere*—first, do no harm.

Hospitals have not been ignoring the problem—far from it. Spurred on by a consumer-driven patient safety movement, they have undertaken hundreds of programs to combat HAI, providing a classic example of the translation of medical research findings into clinical practice and better care for the patient. And the programs have had an impact: The Centers for Disease Control and Prevention (CDC) infection and fatality figures previously cited are considerably lower than earlier estimates. Specifically, in a national point prevalence study applying the CDC's HAI definitions in approximately 200 hospitals, 3% of patients had HAIs in 2015 compared to 4% in 2011 using the same research methods,[3] primarily due to reductions in surgical site infections and urinary tract infections. More recent national data published using hospital-reported National Healthcare Safety Network data for changes reported between 2017 and 2018 indicated central line–associated bloodstream infection (CLABSI) had decreased 9% overall and 11% in the ICU; catheter-associated urinary tract infection (CAUTI) had decreased 8% overall and 10% in the ICU; and hospital-onset *Clostridioides difficile* (formerly known as *Clostridium difficile*) infection (CDI) has decreased 12% overall. However, there has been no significant change in ventilator-associated pneumonia or surgical site infection for the 10 monitored procedures and no change in hospital-onset methicillin-resistant *Staphylococcus aureus* (MRSA) bacteremia.[7]

At one hospital, the scene of a campaign to reduce infections caused by central venous catheters, we interviewed an infection preventionist who wanted to extend the campaign from the ICU to the operating room. At a management Christmas party, over cocktails, he asked the head of anesthesiology whether he was aware that, with the ICU project in full swing, the operating room was now the source of all of the hospital's central venous catheter infections. The anesthesiologist was surprised and chagrined and, in short order, a convert to extending the campaign to his bailiwick.

"My philosophy," the preventionist said, "has always been: What if it's your mother, your father? We always want the best care for those that we love, and we try to bring that home to everyone in the hospital."

But our hospitals as a whole have a long way to go before they realize their infection prevention goals. Although some hospitals do publish successes[6] in prevention of CAUTI and CLABSI in the ICU setting, two recent large collaboratives that focused on ICUs with elevated rates of CLABSI and CAUTI did not demonstrate improved outcomes.[8-10] Overall, reported staff adherence to prevention practices for CLABSI and CAUTI, two of the most common device-related infections, was variable and, in some cases, depressingly low. For CLABSI, reported adherence to prevention policies was nearly 100% for two key recommended practices (maximum sterile barrier precautions during central line insertion and chlorhexidine gluconate for insertion site antisepsis), with adherence to use of chlorhexidine antimicrobial dressing ranging from 86% to 92%. The use of antimicrobial catheters, however, ranged from just 36% to 45%.[11] For CAUTI, though large improvements in key preventive practices were seen compared to the prior 2017 assessment, there remains much room for improvement in basic preventive strategies. The use of portable bladder scanners to avoid unnecessary catheterizations, for example, ranged from 69% to 77%. The use of urinary catheter reminders or discontinuation by nurses ranged from 72% to 79%, and just 23% to 31% reported routine use of external condom catheters in men as an alternative to indwelling urinary catheters.[11]

Difficulties with adherence to standard prevention approaches remain, and educational interventions focused on both technical and even socioadaptive strategies to prevent HAIs too often falter. A recent large collaborative funded by the CDC for hospitals struggling with HAI rates provided and deployed HAI-specific self-assessment and educational materials in multiple formats for CAUTI and CLABSI, as well as for two other common HAIs, CDI and MRSA.[8,9,12,13] Though it failed to reduce HAI rates significantly, new tools were developed that may be of interest to hospitals on the journey to reducing HAIs—more detail is provided on this in the chapters to come.

In addition, there have been government initiatives on state and federal levels. In 2009, for example, the Department of Health and Human Services launched a national action plan, increasing its financial support of HAI-related projects and setting 5-year goals for a major reduction of five of the most serious hospital-acquired infections.[14] The Centers for Medicare & Medicaid Services (CMS) has stopped reimbursing hospitals for the extra costs involved in treating a number of hospital infections.[15,16] Starting in 2014, all CMS payments to hospitals "that rank in the lowest-performing quartile of hospital-acquired conditions," including some infections, were reduced by 1%.[17] And CMS requires that hospitals report their infection rates for several HAIs,[18] information that is critical for understanding how best to target such infections.

We (all three authors of this book) have, individually and jointly, closely observed, participated in, and published academic papers about a number of effective efforts to combat hospital infections. Jennifer Meddings, MD, MSc, is an associate professor of internal medicine and pediatrics at the University of Michigan, who has performed several systematic reviews focused on the impact of interventions to prevent CAUTI.[6,19,20] She developed and led a project using the RAND/UCLA Appropriateness Method to develop the Ann Arbor Criteria for urinary catheter use in hospitalized medical patients, as well as the Michigan Appropriate Perioperative Criteria for common procedures in general surgery and orthopedics.[21,22] Vineet Chopra, MD, MSc, is the chief of the Division of Hospital Medicine and associate professor of medicine at the University of Michigan, Ann Arbor. He was the lead author for the 2015 Michigan Appropriateness Guide for Intravenous Catheters (MAGIC) criteria that define when use of a peripherally inserted central catheter is appropriate.[23] Sanjay Saint, MD, MPH, MACP, is the chief of medicine at the VA Ann Arbor Healthcare System and the George Dock professor of medicine at the University of Michigan, Ann Arbor. He was the lead author of the 2016 article[4] in the *New England Journal of Medicine* that detailed the findings of a large-scale collaborative addressing CAUTI in hospitals throughout the United States, which is discussed in more detail in Chapter 3.

Healthcare-associated infections caused by such indwelling devices are especially common—and preventable. They have thus become the leading edge of efforts to combat HAI. In this book, we focus on examples involving two of the most common medical devices: the indwelling urinary catheter and the central venous catheter.

- The indwelling urinary catheter is also known as a Foley. Infections associated with this catheter, known as CAUTI, though generally less dangerous than other conditions, create serious pain and discomfort for patients and are among the most common device-associated infections in the United States. Among the estimated 62,700 healthcare-associated urinary tract infections each year, 62% (38,585) are CAUTIs in US hospitals, based on medical record reviews in 2015.[3]
- The central venous catheter is commonly referred to as a central line. CLABSIs associated with the use of these catheters are life threatening, particularly because these devices remain in the bloodstream for several weeks or more. Among the estimated 83,600 healthcare-associated bloodstream infections in the United States, 73% (61,092) are CLABSIs occurring annually in hospitals, based on 2015 medical record reviews.[3]

  Peripherally inserted central catheters (PICCs) are a unique type of central venous catheter; these are inserted in peripheral veins of the upper arm but terminate in central veins of the chest. They are thus a central line placed through a peripheral vein. PICCs are inserted by specialized vascular access teams at the bedside and are commonly used outside the ICU. As a result of growing PICC use, more complications from central lines now occur outside critical care settings.

"Bundles" of clinical interventions for preventing infection have been developed for both indwelling and central line catheters. Though these interventions vary in their details, they share the common goal of removing the device as soon as possible.

* * *

The infection prevention framework we present in the chapters to come is primarily focused on CAUTI and CLABSI, with later examples describing how lessons learned and challenges related to prevention of CAUTI and CLABSI apply to other HAIs, such as CDI and MRSA, as well as emerging threats such as *Candida auris*.[24] We have chosen CAUTI as our primary focus because hospitals have found CAUTI far more resistant to quality improvement efforts than other infections, particularly in the ICU setting.[4,10] We also believe that the CAUTI prevention framework can serve a larger purpose: as a model for coping with challenges beyond HAIs, including the prevention of falls and antimicrobial stewardship.

In the quotation that opens this chapter, Peter Drucker marvels at the complexity of the hospital as an organization. The CAUTI model can help us unravel some of that complexity and gain a better understanding of hospitals' operations.

Why is a CAUTI prevention framework an apt model for this larger role? Several reasons are the following:

- CAUTI's impact on patients has long been felt throughout the hospital, from the emergency department to the medical–surgical floor to the ICU and from the inpatient rehab unit to the nursing home.
- CAUTI prevention involves a broad spectrum of hospital personnel, including nurses, physicians, infection preventionists, administrators, nursing aides, and microbiologists.
- CAUTI can easily fly under the radar in an environment governed by the rule of rescue, where heart attacks and other life-threatening events trump all else. The same is true of several other hospital-acquired conditions.
- The CAUTI model relies heavily on widely applicable socioadaptive concerns, rather than on technical elements that vary with each target problem. As is true of many other quality improvement efforts, the success of a CAUTI initiative relies on the full engagement of front-line clinicians and on positive communication between nurses and physicians.

The basic framework of the CAUTI model can be used to combat a variety of infections, including those caused by the more than 30 species of the *Staphylococcus* bacteria, commonly referred to as "*Staph.*" These infections range from the mild, such as a simple boil, to the potentially fatal, such as MRSA. The framework is also an appropriate model for preventing "sepsis," which can occur because of the immune system's destructive reaction to an infection. To put it another way, a case of sepsis can happen because a successful infection prevention program did not.

We have chosen the stand-alone hospital as the venue for our discussion of the CAUTI framework rather than a group of hospitals operating as a collaborative. We believe that an infection prevention campaign can be more clearly presented in that context, but we do discuss the collaborative option in detail in Chapter 8.

In the course of our research, we have identified dozens of best practices—reasons why some hospitals have been more successful in preventing infection than others. The strategies and observations, including many of the actual quotations, were drawn from hundreds of interviews of hospital personnel at all levels, conducted through telephone conversations and during site visits to hospitals from Maine to California. Each stage of an infection prevention project is described and analyzed, from the hospital's decision to undertake the campaign to the putting together of a team to lead it to the actual implementation of the campaign on the hospital floor. The barriers to success are many, from nurses who actively resist any change in their routine, to physicians who oppose any kind of new oversight, to administrators who find ways of delaying the delivery of key resources. We suggest concrete techniques to inform the reader's step-by-step, chapter-by-chapter progress toward the goal of a successful—and sustainable—intervention. We also dedicate Chapter 10 to describing how the CAUTI prevention framework might be applied to another, quite different challenge: CDI.

The ultimate aspiration for any hospital, of course, is a culture of clinical excellence. We talked about that with the medical director of a highly rated hospital, who explained his approach to quality initiatives: "We just say it's evidence-based. You cannot refute evidence-based medicine, and that's the way we're going to do things." The initiative might take a while because "You're changing habits," he said, "but we just keep beating on it."

SUGGESTIONS FOR FURTHER READING

Chopra V, Flanders SA, Saint S. The problem with peripherally inserted central catheters. JAMA 2012;308:1527–1528.

This article discusses the advent and promulgation of a new type of central venous catheter, the PICC. As use of the device grew in clinical settings, recognition of the potential harms it can cause were perhaps underappreciated. In this Viewpoint, the authors examine the reasons driving PICC use, potential for harm, and strategies with which to balance benefits and risks in hospitalized settings.

Meddings J, Saint S. Disrupting the life cycle of the urinary catheter. Clin Infect Dis 2011;52:1291–1293.

This editorial commentary breaks down the "life cycle" of the Foley catheter (Step 1, catheter placement; Step 2, catheter care; Step 3, catheter removal; and Step 4, potential catheter replacement) and provides a framework for interventions to prevent CAUTI. There is no silver bullet solution for preventing CAUTI, but the authors simplify steps that may be taken to decrease infection rates, such as identifying unnecessary catheter use, ensuring sterile placement, maintaining awareness of catheter existence, and seeking prompt removal. This life cycle was adapted by this research team in a subsequent publication[6] to emphasize the need to put a larger focus on avoidance of initial catheter use as Step 0.

Pronovost P, Needham D, Berenholtz S, et al. An intervention to decrease catheter-related bloodstream infections in the ICU. N Engl J Med 2006;355:2725–2732.

In this cohort study of 103 ICUs in Michigan, Pronovost and colleagues found that an evidence-based intervention resulted in a decreased rate of catheter-related bloodstream infection per 1,000 catheter-days, from 2.7 infections at baseline to 0 infections at 3 months postimplementation, and the mean rate per 1,000 catheter-days decreased from 7.7 at baseline to 1.4 at 16 to 18 months of follow-up.

Saint S, Howell JD, Krein SL. Implementation science: how to jump-start infection prevention. Infect Control Hosp Epidemiol 2010;31(suppl 1):S14–S17.

By suggesting a conceptual framework and other key strategies for translating infection prevention evidence into practice, the authors explore infection prevention as a paradigm for implementation science.

Saint S, Meddings JA, Calfee D, Kowalski CP, Krein SL. Catheter-associated urinary tract infection and the Medicare rule changes. Ann Intern Med 2009;150:877–884.

This article explores the 2008 changes in reimbursement by CMS as they apply to CAUTI. The authors provide an overview of CAUTI prevention and the rule changes, as well as suggesting consequences, practical implications, and next steps for hospitals.

Committing to an Infection Prevention Initiative

I think one's feelings waste themselves in words; they ought all to be distilled into actions which bring results.

—Florence Nightingale

"Everyone is interested in quality," the hospital epidemiologist said, explaining why her hospital's leaders had supported an initiative to combat infection, "but the reason behind the interest in quality is not because we're incredibly nice people. It's because if you don't save money, you're going to be bankrupt."

Of course, it's never quite that simple. Like every organization run by human beings, hospitals make decisions in response to a wide variety of carrots and sticks. Financial incentives are an important factor but are far from the only ones. And what makes the equation even more complex is how individual hospitals differ from each other because of such factors as their size, the nature of their patient population, and (there it is again) their financial circumstances.

Along with those factors, though, and influenced by them, is a hospital's level of commitment to excellence in patient care. Over the last few decades, to an important degree, that level of commitment has come to be defined by a hospital's willingness to undertake infection prevention initiatives. Such interventions have saved thousands of patients' lives and saved millions more from various kinds of misery. But the infection threat has grown worse.

Multidrug-resistant organisms (MDROs) are proliferating around the globe. Hospitals' infection prevention efforts—such as those reducing the use of indwelling catheters—keep deadly MDROs like methicillin-resistant *Staphylococcus aureus* (MRSA) out of the bloodstream, and they eliminate the need to use and overuse antimicrobials. Thus, hospital leaders may also approve infection prevention interventions because of the threat that infection poses to their patients; the C-suite actually does house a number of "incredibly nice people."

WHY HOSPITALS SIGN ON

In this chapter, we explore the reasons that hospital officials take on infection prevention initiatives and how they get the ball rolling.

Sometimes the infection prevention decision is part of a package, a larger systems redesign. Many hospitals have adopted a Lean or a Six Sigma approach aimed at improving overall operational efficiency to reduce cost and improve clinical care. Hospital chief executive officers (CEOs) recognize that forestalling infection is eminently efficient as well as humane.

In other cases, CEOs call for an infection prevention intervention because they learn that their hospital's infection rate has been rising above the national norm—or above the rate achieved by nearby competitors. Hospitals in the same area compete for customers—or "patients," as we call them—at least as energetically as any neighborhood stores. They can't afford to fall behind. And now that hospitals' infection rates, along with other measures, have become a matter of public knowledge—via the Centers for Medicare & Medicaid Services' (CMS) Hospital Compare website, for example, and some state websites—administrators have a powerful new motivation for keeping up with the Joneses. The list of healthcare-associated infections (HAIs) publicly reported on Hospital Compare is often evolving, and as of September 2019, this list has included catheter-associated urinary tract infection (CAUTI), central line-associated bloodstream infection (CLABSI), MRSA blood infections, *Clostridium difficile* (now *Clostridioides difficile*), and select surgical site infections (SSIs).[1] A claim to being a town's "safest hospital" can be a powerful marketing tool. By the same token, many a CEO has gotten religion about infection prevention when the hospital down the street announced plans for a major quality initiative or agreed to join in a statewide collaborative project to lower infection rates. As we discuss in Chapter 8, collaboratives—and other safety-focused initiatives, such as high-reliability training programs[2-5]— can exert a powerful magnetic force on a hospital, even though they typically force the staff to jump through any number of hoops.

The impetus for an intervention may also come from within the institution: An intensive care physician returns from an Institute for Healthcare Improvement conference touting the benefits of a new twist on CLABSI prevention or the critical care oversight committee develops a proposal for an intervention to reduce the incidence of CAUTI. Sometimes the genesis of an initiative arises from the ranks of hospital employees, from someone like a nurse we interviewed, a specialist in placing the peripherally inserted central catheter (PICC).

She described her reaction after learning of her hospital's sky-high CLABSI rate: "I was literally crying, tearing my hair out," she said. She asked herself, "What can I do?"

She began by convincing her supervisor to give her an assistant so she would have time to teach nurses at the bedside how to better care for all types of central lines. She focused on the simple things: checking to make sure that dressings were intact, that the line was still being used and thus necessary, and that practices such as flushing or injecting through the line were being performed in a clean and sterile fashion. She lobbied for protected time to research CLABSI prevention and began introducing evidence-based measures to combat the infection. After her campaign was brought to the attention of the hospital's leadership, her prevention approach was adopted in all the hospital's intensive care units (ICUs), and central line infection rates plummeted from 4 per 1,000 catheter days to 1.2.

More typically, an infection prevention intervention starts with the infection prevention staff. They are the people, after all, who collect, analyze, and interpret a hospital's infection data and report the results to hospital personnel and local, state, and federal authorities. They are the first to see negative trends developing in a hospital and among the first to learn about new scientific prevention developments.

Hospital leaders lean toward infection prevention initiatives when the moves are backed by science. An infection preventionist, describing how he presents a proposal for an initiative to management, told us, "We really work at providing evidence-based practices as opposed to, 'This is the new gadget out there; we should go with it.'" And the leadership responds to appeals to patient safety, as well as the potential for reducing hospital costs—typical reimbursement for HAIs does not cover the expenses of caring for patients who develop these infections. Calculators are now available for estimating the cost of CAUTI or CLABSI to individual hospitals, as well as the projected costs of possible interventions to reduce catheter use (see Box 2.1).

However, one of the biggest sticks among the carrots and sticks that influence CEOs is wielded by the federal government, and it carries a larger dollar sign—financial penalties hospitals endure because of excessive rates of healthcare-associated complications, including CAUTI and CLABSI.

LINKING VALUE TO PAYMENT

Since 2008, several policies have been initiated in the United States related to hospital payment by Medicare involving hospital-acquired infections. These policies share the goal of "linking value to payment" by motivating hospitals to reduce both hospital-acquired infections and overall spending by Medicare. The CMS decision to stop reimbursing hospitals in the United States for the extra cost of HAIs, joined in by commercial insurers, has given the C-suite a powerful extra incentive to fight those infections. In this section, we briefly review the major value-based purchasing programs in the United States related to hospital-acquired infections. Although

Box 2.1

CALCULATING COSTS OF CAUTI AND CLABSI

Two online calculator tools are available to estimate an individual hospital's costs related to CAUTI and CLABSI; the websites were developed by the authors and associates at the VA Ann Arbor Healthcare System and the University of Michigan.

- An online calculator tool to help estimate the cost of CAUTI to your hospital is available at **https://www.catheterout.org/cauti-cost-calculator.html.** This calculator can also be used to estimate the projected cost savings following a hypothetical intervention to reduce Foley use.
- An online calculator tool to help estimate the cost of CLABSI, as well as the cost related to venous thromboembolism related to the common PICC, is available at **https://www.improvepicc.com/clabsi-cost-calculator.html.** This calculator can also be used to estimate the projected cost savings following a hypothetical intervention to reduce PICC-related complications by prioritizing the use of devices with fewer lumens.

these policies intermittently are updated to include additional hospital-acquired infections, public reporting requirements, or changes in the size of the payment changes, these policies remain in effect in 2021.

Prior to the October 2008 enforcement of Hospital-Acquired Conditions Initiative,[6] a Medicare inpatient at a large academic hospital with pneumonia would have yielded a CMS payment of $6,072 if there were no complications or comorbidities that would qualify for additional payment; $8,346 if there was also a CAUTI; and $11,891 if there was a more serious complication such as a renal abscess associated with a urinary catheter.[7] Now, because of the Hospital-Acquired Conditions Initiative,[6] CMS pays just the initial $6,072 (in 2008 dollars), and the hospital must absorb the difference. However, there was limited financial impact of this policy on the hospitals,[8] with no significant reductions in CLABSI or CAUTI seen clinically in a large study of these infections as reported to the National Healthcare Safety Network (NHSN),[9] though there was an abrupt drop in billing for these now nonpayable diagnoses.[10] An important reason for this could have been the complex requirements of accurately describing a hospital-acquired CLABSI or CAUTI using diagnosis codes in claims data to trigger removal of the infection as a potentially payable comorbidity,[11] and that if the patient had other comorbidities besides the infection that qualified for extra payment, then no decrease in hospital payment occurred.

However, a survey of infection preventionists,[12] published in 2012, found that 81% of respondents had observed a greater focus since 2008 on the infections targeted by CMS, and nearly 70% were spending more time educating staff on best practices to prevent CLABSI and CAUTI. The survey also discovered that about 50% of respondents said they were spending more time working with physicians and coders to document infections that were present on a patient's *admission* to the hospital. No point in getting stung for infections that occurred before the patient even arrived!

There are, in fact, some serious concerns about how CMS decides these reimbursements, especially its use of "claims"—sometimes referred to as "administrative"—data generated from physicians' notes. Those notes rarely contain the text that coders require to label a urinary tract infection as catheter associated or hospital acquired in billing data. The rate of CAUTI claims is, therefore, much lower than epidemiological studies and surveillance data suggest it should be.[11,12,13] We believe that claims data are not valid for imposing the CMS penalties on HAI or for comparing hospitals in public reporting for healthcare-associated complication rates. Hospitals with higher complication rates in claims data may simply be better at documenting those conditions or have a patient population more susceptible to infection.

Fortunately, a recent decision from the federal government addresses these issues. Since October 1, 2014, quality measures and scoring methodology related to HAIs have been improved, no longer relying on claims data alone, specifically for CLABSI and CAUTI rates. Rather than base rates on claims data, the CMS now uses the NHSN database for measuring most HAI rates, including CLABSI and CAUTI for comparing hospital performance for public reporting on Medicare's Hospital Compare website.[1] The NHSN database surveillance data collection begins with hospital reports of positive cultures, such as positive urine and blood cultures, in which infection preventionists at the hospital review the chart for qualifying catheter use and symptoms by applying NHSN definitions for CLABSI and CAUTI.[14] NHSN rates for public reporting and comparing hospital performance are standardized to adjust for various facility-level factors that contribute to HAI risk within each unit, but they do not account for comorbidities of individual patients that develop the HAIs.[15]

However, note that the NHSN system was designed as a surveillance system, not for identifying clinical infections for penalizing hospitals. Like any good surveillance system, it tries to balance sensitivity and specificity to screen in potential cases—not just positive ones. Therefore, there are ongoing discussions of how to improve or replace this system to optimally identify clinically significant HAIs and ideas for how to replace manual chart review by infection preventionists for qualifying signs and symptoms with automated data extraction from electronic medical records.

Two other major CMS[16,17] programs were later implemented in the United States to further support the goal of reducing payment to hospitals with elevated rates of HAIs. Since the October 2014 implementation of the Hospital-Acquired Condition Reduction Program (HACRP),[16] hospitals are compared nationally by a composite score (called the Patient Safety Indicator [PSI] 90) that includes rates of several hospital-acquired conditions as documented in claims data, as well as rates of several infections, such as CLABSI and CAUTI, as reported by hospitals to the NHSN. Hospitals with a total composite hospital-acquired conditions score from claims data and NHSN data in the worst quartile of performance nationwide then are penalized by a 1% reduction in payment applied to all Medicare discharges that year for the hospital. Similarly, the Hospital Value-Based Purchasing Program[17] implemented in 2012 also compares hospital performance by many metrics, including the same CAUTI, CLABSI, and PSI-90 measures reported in the Hospital-Acquired Condition Reduction Program (HACRP) and uses 2% of usual Medicare payment to these hospitals "at risk" to then later reward hospitals that had better performance. Data conflict whether these two programs have stimulated improvements in patient outcomes and healthcare spending conflicts, as it varies by the years compared, type of data used for analysis, and definitions.[18]

Analyses of NHSN surveillance data from 2006 to 2018 indicate that both CLABSI and CAUTI have declined over time, with CLABSI having faster declines in earlier years (approximately 50% reduction from 2008 to 2016) than CAUTI, with CAUTI reductions occurring more steadily only in recent years after a major definition change in 2015, with the removal of yeast as a qualifying microbe for CAUTI definition.[19] Annual reductions in NHSN rates between 2015 and 2018 have varied from 9% to 11% for CLABSI and 5% to 8% for CAUTI.[20] Substantial reductions in mortality and costs were reported in analysis of CLABSI and CAUTI events as recorded in the Medicare Patient Safety Monitoring System (comparing 2011–2014 data with 2010 data), which is a surveillance system that identifies adverse events like CLABSI and CAUTI from chart review of randomly selected Medicare inpatients using somewhat different definitions of catheter use and qualifying symptoms than the NHSN definitions.[21] Additionally, a recent analysis involving a multistate point prevalence medical record review of HAI rates supported that there was a significant reduction in the percentage of patients with CAUTI in 2015 (0.20 with 95% confidence interval [CI] 0.13–0.29) compared to 2011 (0.39, 95% CI 0.29–0.52); however, there was no significant reduction in the percentage of patients with CLABSI between 2015 (0.37, 95% CI 0.27–0.50) and 2011 (0.30, 95% CI 0.22–0.42).[22] Of note, the concept of publicly reporting hospital performance and/or penalizing based on hospital-acquired complication rates such as hospital-acquired infections or process measures related to infection prevention is also gradually gaining support outside the United States, including programs in the United Kingdom, Australia, and Canada.[23-26]

Though financial matters loom large in a hospital's decision to initiate an infection prevention program, they are not alone. A major factor is the nature of the institutional culture. Is the hospital fully committed to quality patient care as its core mission? Does that concern for the patient weigh heavily in the leaders' major decisions?

In the course of our research, we found a large public hospital that came close to meeting those standards. The fact that the staff served a largely poverty-stricken patient population actually seemed to nurture such a patient-centered approach.

"There's a bunch of homeless folks that come here," the chief of staff told us, "so it's a real 'get-down-and-get-dirty' kind of place. But everybody loves to be here, whether you're in OB or you're psych or you're peds, because they get a chance to make a difference in peoples' lives."

A quality manager at this hospital added that the staff had to be "as nice as we can be to some people who aren't very nice to us, so it just takes a special kind of person to be down here, and I think that's why it works."

The chief executive officer, staff members told us, was another essential element in the hospital's success, in part because she is a nurse with a deep understanding of what happens on the patient floors and in part because of her patient-centered, collaborative management style. Several people described the culture of the hospital as "collegial" and "egalitarian." Nurses serve on all of the medical staff committees, and all the other committees have doctor members. The chief of staff described the workings of the critical care committee, which he said includes doctors, nurses, and "everybody else." For things to happen, he went on, requires agreement across the board: "It's like an end-of-life discussion where the decision is made with everybody on the same page."

This is the same institution that was mobilized by the vascular access lead nurse to undertake the program to prevent CLABSI. What counted was not the source of the idea but its validity as a means of improving patient care.

When we asked that hospital's epidemiologist about his institution's culture, he replied, "Striving for excellence would be a fair way to describe it." That's also a fair description of the model hospital that will be making a regular appearance in the chapters to come. This midsize, 250-bed facility, an entity entirely of our own invention, is intended to serve as a framework on which to hang dozens of infection prevention best practices.

To be sure, for any given challenge, there are all sorts of potential solutions that may be better or worse, depending on the particular circumstances and the nature of the particular hospital and its staff. We will present a host of such solutions along the way, but we also want to provide a coherent, step-by-step picture of how a successful infection prevention initiative might be conducted—starting with the decision to proceed.

THE CEO MAKES A DECISION

At the model hospital, that decision has been generated at the top. The CEO, cognizant of the CMS pressure on the financial side and the need to reduce infections, consults with his clinical leaders. They agree to take on a small package of initiatives covering CAUTI and CLABSI prevention.

The next question is, who, from among the leadership, is going to oversee each initiative? The project sponsor has to be willing and able to take on this extra responsibility. It is not likely to consume all that much of his or her time, but there will be some initial meetings and a steady stream of reports to look over. A project manager will have to be found to be the operational leader. And the sponsor will be called on if and when the initiative triggers disputes or problems that cannot be resolved in the lower ranks.

At the model hospital, the CEO and the chief of staff (otherwise known as the chief medical officer or vice president of medical affairs) call in the director of critical care for a heart-to-heart talk. They urge him to accept executive sponsorship of the CAUTI and CLABSI initiatives that will be focused in the hospital's two ICUs, one medical and the other surgical. The director points out that the interventions will require some major changes in practice that could strain his department's budget, but in the end, he agrees to take on the extra job. In any event, he expects the nurses and physicians in charge of each ICU to run their own programs.

The CEO turns the CAUTI initiative over to the chief nursing executive since it calls for a change in the hospital's bedside nursing practice. With her top deputy, the director of nursing, the chief nursing executive goes over a list of potential sponsors, including the head of quality and the chief infection preventionist. The head of quality, they decide, is too academic, too removed from the problems of the wards and unlikely to be viewed as an effective change agent. The infection preventionist, although she has a solid reputation among both physicians and nurses, has no experience in bedside nursing care. They know that in order to get buy-in from the floor nurses, it will be imperative to have someone who has "walked the talk." The chief nurse finally urges her deputy, the director of nursing, to become the project's executive sponsor—and receives the answer she hoped for.

In her role as executive sponsor, the director of nursing understands that even though the CAUTI initiative has the support of the hospital's leaders, they have many other concerns—projects and challenges that may have a higher priority. She knows that she will probably have to battle to obtain extra funding for some aspects of the intervention, primarily new products like portable ultrasounds and perhaps even overtime as nurses struggle to learn a new way of dealing with indwelling catheters. They will be following a checklist of behaviors embodied in the bladder bundle, an evidence-based collection of do's and don'ts (see Box 2.2).

If the model hospital runs true to form, the executive sponsor realizes there will be plenty of staff opposition to the ICU intervention. The history of quality improvement is filled with tales of people, set in their ways, who ridiculed such changes as the presurgery time-out until it saved them from embarrassing error. Now a standard of care, the time-out requires the verbal identification of every aspect of the procedure from the names of the patient and participants to the name of the procedure and its location on the patient.

More recently, many hospitals have encountered a refusal by a substantial percentage of their staff to obey hand hygiene rules, despite proven efficacy. Some hospitals have installed elaborate technological aids to

Box 2.2

RECOMMENDATIONS FOR PREVENTING CATHETER-ASSOCIATED
URINARY TRACT INFECTION "*ABCDE*"[a]

- *A*septic catheter insertion and proper maintenance are paramount.
- *B*ladder ultrasound may avoid indwelling catheterization.
- *C*ondom catheters or other alternatives to an indwelling catheter such as intermittent catheterization should be considered in appropriate patients.
- *D*o not use the indwelling catheter unless you must!
- *E*arly removal of the catheter using a reminder or nurse-initiated removal protocol when it appears warranted.

[a]Adapted from Saint et al.[27]

check up on staff adherence to the rules. In one example, a video camera records whether people entering an intensive care room wash their hands. In another example, staffers wear badges that vibrate when they approach a patient's bed if they have failed to wash their hands. To outwit the devices, some hidebound staffers have ducked under waist-high monitors and turned on the water in the room's sink to avoid a badge reaction but without washing their hands.[28]

At the model hospital, the executive sponsor is happily aware that she will not personally have to impose a new Foley procedure on the staff. That will be the task of the project manager and his or her team, including a nurse champion and a physician champion. The sponsor will have to find a project manager, who will, in turn, assemble the team.

The sponsor actually has a candidate in mind, one of her own—a veteran unit manager who has put together a model inpatient nursing unit. She is assertive when necessary, and she knows what buttons to push. She also has a full measure of the needed interpersonal skills: She is patient, persistent, and enthusiastic about improving patient care, and she has built positive relationships with many of the hospital's nurses and physicians in the course of managing previous quality initiatives. Before the sponsor talks with her, though, she consults with the chief nursing executive, winning her approval.

In the chapters ahead, our description of the model hospital will mainly focus on its CAUTI prevention effort as a best-practice example, although we also weave in and discuss the particular personnel challenges of initiatives to reduce CLABSI and *Clostridioides difficile* infection (CDI). Our goal throughout is to offer field-tested insights to aid in the adoption and implementation of quality improvement initiatives.

SUGGESTIONS FOR FURTHER READING

Burke JP. Infection control—a problem for patient safety. N Engl J Med 2003;348: 651–656.

In this article, Burke discusses the major problems in infection control, approaches for solving these problems, the role of the National Nosocomial Infections Surveillance System of the Centers for Disease Control and Prevention (precursor to the current NHSN system) as a model, and the need for renewed commitment to, and innovations in, infection control to help ensure patient safety. This was one of the first articles that linked infection prevention and control to patient safety.

Krein SL, Greene MT, Apisarnthanarak A, et al. Infection prevention practices in Japan, Thailand, and the United States: results from national surveys. Clin Infect Dis 2017;64:S105–S111.

Data from hospital surveys across Japan, Thailand, and the United States were analyzed in this study to determine the use of recommended practices to prevent common device-associated infections, as well as to identify hospital characteristics associated with the use of select practices. Regular use of practices to prevent CLABSI and VAP were reported among the majority of hospitals from all three countries, while CAUTI prevention practices were variable, with fewer practices adopted.

Meddings J, McMahon LF, Jr. Web exclusives. Annals for hospitalists inpatient notes— legislating quality to prevent infection—a primer for hospitalists. Ann Intern Med 2017;166:HO2–HO3.

This commentary tackles three major Medicare policies intended to target rates of CAUTI and CLABSI in the hospital to improve safety while promoting Medicare savings. The authors point out that while these programs successfully reduce Medicare spending, it is unclear whether they have impacted clinical care. The ideal future of these complex programs is that they would be informed by front-line physicians so they are effective in reducing infection rates and advancing patient safety.

Saint S, Greene MT, Fowler KE, et al. What US hospitals are currently doing to prevent common device-associated infections: results from a national survey. BMJ Qual Saf 2019;28:741–749.

In this study, infection preventionists across the nation were surveyed regarding their use of practices to prevent common device-associated infections, including CAUTI, CLABSI, and ventilator-associated pneumonia (VAP). Ninety percent of the surveyed hospitals reported use of several practices. Among the top practices currently used in US hospitals were aseptic technique during indwelling urethral catheter insertion and maintenance and maximum sterile barrier precautions during central catheter insertion with alcohol-containing chlorhexidine gluconate for insertion site antisepsis.

Saint S, Lipsky BA, Goold SD. Indwelling urinary catheters: a one-point restraint? Ann Intern Med 2002;137:125–127.

In this editorial, the authors discuss the often unjustified and excessively prolonged persistence of urinary catheter use despite clear evidence of its detrimental effects. They discuss the practical effect of needlessly confining patients in what could be called a "one-point" restraint, raising serious safety and ethical concerns analogous to those noted more than a decade ago with "four-point" (limb) restraints; they propose that lessons learned from efforts to curtail the use of physical restraints may help identify strategies for diminishing the use of indwelling urinary catheters.

Umscheid CA, Mitchell MD, Doshi JA, Agarwal R, Williams K, Brennan PJ. Estimating the proportion of healthcare-associated infections that are reasonably preventable and the related mortality and costs. Infect Control Hosp Epidemiol 2011;32:101–114.

In this study, Umscheid and colleagues performed a systematic review of interventions to reduce HAIs and national data to estimate the preventability of CLABSI, CAUTI, VAP, and SSI. They found that as many as 65% to 70% of cases of CLABSI and CAUTI and 55% of cases of VAP and SSI may be preventable with current evidence-based strategies. These results suggest that, although 100% prevention may be unattainable, comprehensive implementation of evidence-based strategies could prevent hundreds of thousands of infections and save tens of thousands of lives and billions of dollars.

Types of Interventions

Catheter-Associated Urinary Tract Infection

The great tragedy of science is the slaying of a beautiful hypothesis
by an ugly fact.

—THOMAS HENRY HUXLEY

Long before there were hospitals, there were healthcare-associated
infections (HAIs), contracted in the course of self-treatment. There
has, for example, always been some kind of urinary catheter that a
person might use to cope with urinary incontinence and other such
difficulties—and some kind of urinary tract infection as a result. In this
chapter addressing catheter-associated urinary tract infection (CAUTI),
and the following chapter, targeting central line–associated bloodstream
infection (CLABSI), our focus is on the basics of infection prevention
and current best practices. In each chapter, we describe a two-tiered
approach for prioritizing interventions as well as an online assessment
tool known as the Guide to Patient Safety (GPS) tailored to each kind
of infection. But first, a bit of important background on the history of
hospital-acquired infections and lessons learned from early trials of infection prevention.

HOSPITALS AND THE GERM THEORY OF DISEASE

For many millions of people, suffering from urinary retention or incontinence or recovering from genitourinary surgery, the catheter can be a godsend. But like any foreign object introduced into the body, be it a central venous catheter or an endotracheal tube attached to a mechanical ventilator, the urinary catheter can introduce or serve as a reservoir of infection. The effort to prevent the infections that can arise because of these objects, the subject of this book, is part of a larger, long-running campaign to stave off infection in the hospital setting.

A major milestone in that effort came in the 1840s when a Viennese physician, Ignaz Semmelweis, discovered the cause of a flare-up of puerperal fever in a delivery room. The medical students who were helping with deliveries often arrived in the room directly from performing autopsies— and without properly washing their hands. Once they began washing with a chlorinated lime solution, the death rate in the maternity ward plunged by 500%! When Semmelweis sought to spread word of his discovery, he was ridiculed and forced from his position. In a new post at a different hospital, he confirmed his findings, but the powers that be in the healthcare community still rejected his ideas. He eventually became emotionally unstable and died in an insane asylum at the age of 47.

The resistance of the medical profession to change, even such a simple and well-confirmed change, may seem startling in retrospect. And yet, here we are, more than a century and a half later, still struggling to convince hospital personnel to wash their hands regularly. In spite of a full-press international campaign, average hand hygiene rates are only about 40%.[1]

The prevailing wisdom in Semmelweis's time held that disease was spread by foul-smelling and poisonous vapors, miasmas, caused by the rotting of organic substances. Cholera, for example, was thought to be caused by breathing in bad air or drinking contaminated water. Enter Louis Pasteur, the 19th-century French chemist who so famously proved otherwise.

At the time, the process that created wine, beer, and vinegar was thought to be a simple chemical reaction producing yeast as a byproduct. Pasteur showed that, in fact, microorganisms, in this case yeast, were responsible for the fermentation process, and he succeeded in identifying the germs that sometimes fouled the process—producing sour milk or reducing alcohol production. He further discovered that he could kill these destructive germs by heating them—the process we call pasteurization.

If germs could cause fermentation, Pasteur thought, perhaps they might cause infectious diseases as well. Eventually, that led him to confirm the germ theory of disease. It holds that pathogens such as viruses and bacteria, unseeable to the naked eye, invade human and animal hosts and give rise to infectious diseases. The acceptance of the germ theory would forever transform the practice of medicine, and the theory's link with the laboratory would confer on physicians the imprimatur of science. It remains the bedrock premise of modern medicine and medical research.

In the 1860s, Joseph Lister, a Glasgow surgeon, was an interested reader of Pasteur's work, in particular a paper suggesting that heat, filtration, or exposure to chemicals might be used to kill the germs that caused gangrene. Lister tested this hypothesis by spraying carbolic acid on surgical instruments and incisions, thereby vastly reducing postoperative gangrene.

THE HISTORY OF INFECTION CONTROL

With the growing acceptance of the germ theory, hospitals increasingly used isolation to prevent the transmission of infectious diseases, and sanitary conditions in general improved, but hospitals continued to be breeding grounds for infection. Infectious diseases physicians and microbiologists gradually began to specialize in infection prevention, and a handful of hospitals developed infection control programs in the 1950s. Public health agencies initially kept their hands off, apparently believing that hospitals had the wherewithal to cure themselves, but in 1965, the Centers for Disease Control and Prevention (CDC) did make a major contribution to infection prevention with the creation of the Comprehensive Hospital Infections Project. Eight community hospitals around the United States were chosen to function as CDC laboratories for the study of HAI epidemiology and the development of infection prevention techniques. The National Nosocomial Infections Surveillance System (NNIS) was established in 1970 to routinely collect hospital-acquired infection surveillance data for aggregation into a national database. In 2005, the CDC decided to combine the NNIS with the National Surveillance System for Healthcare Workers, a merger that included the Dialysis Surveillance Network, which the CDC had been separately managing under its Division of Healthcare Quality Promotion. Thus, the National Healthcare Safety Network (NHSN), a comprehensive system for the tracking of HAIs, was born. Starting with 300 hospitals, the network now gathers infection data from more than 11,000 medical facilities, including acute and postacute care settings.

As infection control gained traction in hospitals, it became a potential new career path for staff members, including nurses, microbiologists, and infectious diseases physicians, which in turn gave fresh impetus to the infection control movement. In 1972, they gained a professional society with the founding of the Association of Practitioners in Infection Control (APIC), now the Association for Professionals in Infection Control and Epidemiology, and other more specialized professional societies soon followed. These groups helped provide the trained professionals the infection prevention movement required to effectively reduce infections in US hospitals.

Despite these signs of progress, the CDC was not satisfied with the state of HAI prevention. As a result, the agency initiated a national study in 1974 now known as the Study on the Effectiveness of Nosocomial Infection Control (the SENIC Project). The study found that only about half of the 338 hospitals examined had infection surveillance and control systems, but those with such systems in place had substantially lower rates of HAI. That result convinced the Joint Commission on Accreditation of Hospitals to require, as of 1976, that hospitals must operate CDC-recommended infection prevention programs to maintain their accreditation.

Yet HAI was still an afterthought when the Institute of Medicine published a watershed study in 1999, "To Err Is Human." It inspired widespread media coverage, putting patient safety in general on the public agenda, but it accorded HAI just five paragraphs—and even that in an appendix to the main report. Infection prevention leaders, however, were able to ride the patient safety wave, alerting the public to the extensive and harmful impact of HAI. Their efforts led to the passage of state laws requiring hospitals to publicly report their infection rates. The theory was that this exposure of medical error would help spur hospitals to greater efforts to prevent infection.

Since then, HAI has become a major component of the national and international movement to enhance patient safety. Almost a third of the hospital-acquired conditions that the Centers for Medicare & Medicaid Services no longer reimburses are HAIs. About half of the initiatives in the Institute for Healthcare Improvement's 100,000 Lives campaign were concerned with infection prevention.

The infection prevention movement has come of age within the public health community. And our understanding of the technical side of prevention has made great strides, which will become evident, we trust, in the pages just ahead as we describe the bundles of interventions behind CAUTI and CLABSI prevention. The greater challenge, the struggle to win the active support of the clinical staff for these prevention initiatives, the adaptive challenge, is described in the following chapters.

CATHETER-ASSOCIATED URINARY TRACT INFECTION

Urinary catheterization has a storied past. The ancient Chinese relied on onion stalks to pass through the urethra into the bladder to release urine because of the dysfunction of nerves or muscles or a blockage. The ancient Egyptians and Greeks used tubes of wood and metal. Benjamin Franklin invented a flexible catheter in 1752 to relieve his brother, John, who had bladder stones, and probably used it somewhat later on himself for the same problem. During the 1930s, Dr. Frederic Eugene Basil Foley was one of several urologists who were developing catheters that had a small, water-inflated balloon on the end that kept the device from slipping out of the body. Eventually, the indwelling balloon catheter was universally adopted, and it was Dr. Foley's name that became permanently attached to the device.

The popularity of the indwelling urinary catheter today is impressive. More than 100 million Foleys are used each year, worldwide, and US hospitals account for more than a quarter of them. Foleys are often convenient, for medical staff and for some patients. The use of an indwelling catheter avoids the need for toileting patients and requires only that the bag that collects urine be emptied when necessary.

Foleys are not, however, universally popular. One study[2] found that 42% of catheterized patients said the Foley was uncomfortable, 48% said it was painful, and 61% said it restricted their activities of daily living. It can serve as a one-point restraint, binding patients to their beds, which promotes such complications as venous thromboembolism and pressure ulcers. And if the Foley's balloon is not completely deflated on removal, it can cause severe damage to the urinary tract. Catheterization can also delay patients' departure from a hospital if they cannot void normally following the Foley's removal.

The most important black mark against the Foley, though, is that it causes about 70% of all hospital-associated urinary tract infections.[3] CAUTIs are one of the most common of all hospital infections. The longer the catheter remains in the body, the greater the chance that bacteria will travel up from the bag during routine maintenance of the Foley or any manipulation of the device.

At the model hospital we introduced in the previous chapter, the initiative to reduce CAUTI relies on a so-called bladder bundle, a combination of best practices, equipment, and protocols. Research by behavioral scientists has shown that the odds of success in infection control programs are improved by focusing on several modes of intervention rather than just one or two. That is not to say, however, that hospitals should take a multimodal-or-nothing approach; a more narrowly focused intervention is better than none.

The basic message of the bladder bundle is this: Don't use the Foley unless it's really necessary—and if you do use it, regularly reassess whether its use is still indicated so it is removed as soon as possible.

The bundle at our model hospital includes the following:

- Hand hygiene by clinicians while inserting the catheter and each time the catheter is touched for care or emptying. Use soap and water or an alcohol-based cleanser.

- A standardized kit containing a Foley with presealed junctions to prevent bacteria from entering the system, along with drapes and all other items to ensure an aseptic insertion with securement and a properly functioning catheter. Given a recent study[4] documenting breaks in aseptic insertion technique in 48 (59%) of 81 observed urinary catheter insertions in an emergency room, clinicians should consider including an additional set of clinician hands to help with patient instructions and positioning, as well as lighting and assistance with tissue retraction if needed to improve visualization of the urethral meatus.

- A urinary management policy that sets forth appropriate and inappropriate indications for the use of Foleys. The RAND/ UCLA Appropriateness Method,[5] which combines systematic literature review as well as formal appropriateness ratings of hundreds of clinical scenarios, clarifies the use of indwelling urinary catheters (i.e., Foley catheters), external catheters, and intermittent straight catheters in hospitalized medical patients; it has been published with open access as the "Ann Arbor Criteria for Appropriate Urinary Catheter Use" in the *Annals of Internal Medicine* (Appendix A, Boxes A.1–A.3, Table A.1, and Figure A.1). For patients undergoing common general surgery and orthopedic surgery procedures, it has been published as the Michigan Appropriate Perioperative Urinary Catheter Criteria in the *BMJ Quality and Safety* (Appendix B, Table B.1). Other criteria for Foley use have been published for appropriate catheter management after surgery for benign prostatic hypertrophy.[6]

Appropriate indications include acute urinary retention or bladder outlet obstruction; the need for accurate measurements of urinary output in critically ill patients; and a number of surgery-related circumstances. Inappropriate indications include using a Foley, instead of standard nursing practice, for urinary incontinence; for assessing urinary output in a patient who is not critically ill; and for obtaining urine for testing when the patient can voluntarily void.

- A standard operating procedure covering Foley insertion, maintenance, and removal. It calls for the use of a nursing assessment template added to the electronic medical record. Appropriate hand hygiene before and after handling the urinary catheter—à la Semmelweis—is also emphasized. Additionally, the protocol requires bedside nurses to make a daily template entry indicating whether any given Foley meets one or more of the appropriate indications for catheter use. If an in-place catheter fails that test, the nurse is to alert the appropriate physician caring for the patient and recommend the catheter's removal. Under a hospital protocol, nurses are empowered by a standing order to remove inappropriate Foleys if there is any substantial delay in obtaining the physician's agreement to the removal.

- Supplies and clinician training to encourage and enable appropriate use of alternatives to Foley catheters. These alternatives include the use of portal bladder ultrasound to verify urinary retention that would benefit from catheterization, intermittent catheterization with a straight catheter (with appropriate indications summarized in Appendix A, Box A.2); external collection devices (with appropriate indications summarized in Appendix A, Box A.3) for men[7] (e.g., condom catheters, glans-adherent catheters) and for women[8,9] (e.g., wicking devices with suction for bed-bound patients with incontinence); and other toileting options, such as a bedpan or bedside commode.[10]

The model hospital also employs two types of reminder systems. The first alerts clinicians to the presence of a Foley catheter so that they can take this into account when making clinical decisions. It reminds doctors and bedside nurses that a Foley is being used for the patient and provides a list of the appropriate reasons to continue or discontinue the catheter. The reminder is included in the patient's medical record— which can be a paper chart (example in Figure 3.1) but at the model hospital is recorded within the patient's electronic medical record. Different versions of this type of reminder include documentation of the presence and/or the duration of a urinary catheter in a printed checklist tool reviewed daily by the clinical team or a visual reminder on a summary page within the electronic medical record, which can be in the form of text in a table of catheter types in use or noted as a symbol on a diagram or figure representing the patient to note the presence of devices such as catheters.

The model hospital, which uses computerized orders, also has the capability of sending an electronic reminder to the physician after a Foley has been in use for 24 or 48 hours, as a way to encourage removal if no longer indicated; a reminder can also be sent to the bedside nurse, who may be empowered to remove the device if it is no longer required for an appropriate clinical indication. Reminders are generally dispatched as a hospital unit eases into an infection prevention initiative to reduce inappropriate urinary catheter use, though care is needed to ensure reminders are directed at the most appropriate clinician on the team for prompting catheter removal while minimizing alarm fatigue as much as possible. Researchers have demonstrated the effectiveness of this type of reminder. One study at a Veterans Health Administration medical center found that the use of a computerized reminder shortened the duration of catheterization by three days while not affecting the rate of recatheterization.[11]

The second type of reminder system used at the model hospital is the stop order. Nurses have been empowered to discontinue the use of a catheter when it is no longer required for an appropriate clinical indication. The stop order tells the patient's bedside nurse to remove an unnecessary

*******URINARY CATHETER REMINDER*******

Date: _____

This patient has had an indwelling urinary catheter since _____

Please indicate below either your 1) approval to remove the catheter **OR** 2) state the reason for continued indwelling urinary catheterization.

☐ Please discontinue indwelling urinary catheter; **OR**

☐ Please continue indwelling urinary catheter because patient requires indwelling catheterization for the following reasons (please check all that apply):

    ☐ Patient has acute urinary retention or bladder outlet obstruction

    ☐ Need for accurate measurements of urinary output in critically ill patients

    ☐ To assist in healing of open sacral or perineal wounds in incontinent patients

    ☐ Patient requires prolonged immobilization (e.g., potentially unstable thoracic or lumbar spine, multiple traumatic injuries such as pelvic fractures)

    ☐ To improve comfort for end of life care if needed

    ☐ Other (please specify): _____

_____   _____
Physician's signature   Doctor number

Figure 3.1 Example of a urinary catheter reminder. (Adapted from Saint et al.[12] and Gould et al.[13])

Foley. The rare exception to the rule is when an additional separate physician order is required if the patient has certain conditions, such as recent urologic surgery.

Both varieties of reminder system have proven their effectiveness. In one analysis of a number of CAUTI studies,[14] the reminders decreased infections by 53%.

NEW APPROACHES TO CAUTI PREVENTION

The distance between our model hospital and the real world is painfully evident in the history of hospitals' CAUTI prevention efforts. In spite of a wide selection of strategies and scores of interventions across the country, so many hospitals have been unable to reduce their CAUTI rates, and it still accounts for almost a third of all acute care hospital infections. In an effort to help hospitals organize and prioritize their infection prevention strategies, a multidisciplinary team from the University of Michigan has developed a tiered approach based on a systematic literature review[15] and expert experience that was a key element of a national initiative financed by the CDC.

The initiative had a mouthful of a name, the States Targeting Reduction in Infections Via Engagement (STRIVE).[16] It sought to bring state organizations together in implementing a curriculum to prevent HAIs at hundreds of hospitals with high HAI rates. The HAIs targeted included CAUTI, CLABSI, *Clostridioides difficile* infection (CDI), and methicillin-resistant *Staphylococcus aureus* bloodstream infection (MRSA bacteremia). Hospitals participating in the year-long implementation were offered monthly webinars and in-person online sessions with feedback. There were also extensive site visits that included coaching. The backbone of the anti-infection curriculum, though, was a series of web-based educational modules organized around a two-tiered approach for prioritizing interventions, including the use of an online assessment tool known as the Guide to Patient safety (GPS), tailored for each infection.

Tier 1 of the CAUTI modules[17] set forth five basic prevention strategies (Appendix C, Figure C.1): (1) using indwelling urinary catheters only when appropriate; (2) finding alternatives to indwelling catheters; (3) ensuring that proper insertion techniques and maintenance procedures are followed; (4) promptly removing unneeded catheters; and (5) requesting urine cultures only when necessary. We have previously discussed the first four strategies. The fifth strategy may still be new to many hospitals and is a critical one. When hospitals order unnecessary urine cultures, it often leads to the inappropriate use of antibiotics to treat normal bacteria that show up in the culture.

Tier 2 (Appendix C, Figure C.1)[17] was intended for hospitals whose infection rates were still elevated after their implementation of the Tier 1 strategies. It offered potential solutions that required greater human and/or material resources. Tier 2 begins with use of the GPS, another tool developed at the University of Michigan. The CAUTI GPS[18-20] consisted of a series of 14 yes/no, self-diagnostic questions aimed at identifying the hospital's particular problems with their CAUTI initiative (Appendix D, Box D.1). Among the questions were the following: Do bedside nurses assess, at least daily, whether their catheterized patients still need a urinary catheter? Have you experienced substantial physician resistance?

The CAUTI GPS then provided a list of enhanced solutions, tailored to each hospital's responses. In addition to the detailed response, the GPS offered links to more extended discussions as well as further reading suggestions. Here are two examples of the GPS at work:

1. If a hospital's answers indicated that it was not routinely giving front-line staff up-to-date data on CAUTI-related matters, the GPS would note that timely and useful feedback to staff could help them stay motivated and engaged in the infection prevention initiative. The enhanced solution would include suggestions about the kinds of data to be shared and the various ways to do it—an infection scorecard to be displayed throughout the hospital, for example, or a newsletter. Another suggestion was to reward a staff member or a unit for positive changes—a photo commemorating the occasion with the chief medical officer or a pizza party for a unit that had brought its high CAUTI rate down to zero.

2. If a hospital indicated that indwelling urinary catheters were commonly being inserted inappropriately in the emergency department (ED), the GPS would note that the nurses and doctors in the ED were more concerned about keeping their patients alive than about whether they needed a catheter. That said, the GPS-enhanced solutions suggested that the CAUTI prevention team include ED department personnel—a physician as well as a nurse—when the initiative moved to the ED, and that the project manager and/or the ED nurse champion spend part of each day walking through the ED, reminding everyone they see about the intervention. Another suggestion was to have the project leader share the latest data on the ED CAUTI-related

performance, including the number of catheters that started out
in the ED, the percentage of them placed inappropriately, and the
percentage that led to infection.

A total of 387 hospitals from 23 states and the District of Columbia
were actively enrolled in the STRIVE project. Among the participants, 250
were acute care hospitals; 76 were critical access; and 35 were long-term
acute care. Most were urban and nonprofit.

Of the total, 361 STRIVE hospitals reported their CAUTI data, which included measures of the CAUTI rate per thousand patients and the number
of catheter days per 100 patients. The results were not impressive.[21] Over
the study period, there were just slight reductions in the two measures. No
substantial quantitative improvements occurred. There were some important caveats to be considered in sizing up the intervention. Even though
STRIVE was designed to target hospitals with high infection rates, a substantial number of hospitals with low rates took part. In fact, the majority
of hospitals participating already had CAUTI rates of 1.0 or lower before
the intervention. In addition, the intervention was brief, with a relatively
short assessment period.

One of the goals of the STRIVE project was to foster relationships
among the hospitals participating as well as such institutions as state hospital associations and state health departments. That goal was achieved,[22]
as noted from phone interviews with participating organizations that
supported personnel from the various groups, and hospitals worked together during the intervention organizing meetings, taking part in advisory calls with hospitals, and conducting site visits.

Some lessons were learned. A University of Michigan team offered
these suggestions for future interventions to improve implementation of
interventions to reduce CAUTI in collaboratives similar to STRIVE:

1. Make sure in advance that hospitals scheduled to engage in a
   web-based intervention have the necessary software.
2. Design the website so that it will track hospitals' record of
   participation in order to feed participation rates back as well

as detect and help troubleshoot difficulties accessing the intervention materials.

3. Increase in-person visits to participating hospitals to monitor and encourage their intervention efforts.

4. Consider providing additional financial resources as part of the collaborative (either from the collaborative's sponsor or by requiring commitment from the participating hospital's C-suite) to encourage and enable specific changes in clinician behavior, such as removing unnecessary devices. These resources could be used to encourage staff to perform tasks that are better for patient care but inconvenient for clinicians—removing indwelling urinary catheters from incontinent patients, for example. Raffle tickets could be offered, with gift certificates, paid time off, or special parking privileges as prizes. Additional unit staff support could be provided for performing the extra bedside tasks of continence care or measuring urine output or weights when indwelling catheters are removed. With such support, unit nurses would be able to undertake such tasks as observing urinary catheter insertions to assess competence or daily reviews of urinary catheter necessity and maintenance care (i.e., "Foley rounds").

WHEN PROOF IS HARD TO FIND

New devices, such as the items in the quality improvement bundles we have been describing, win medical acceptance in part because of their scientific backing. The gold standard in such matters, of course, is the randomized controlled trial in which the study subjects are randomly assigned to one treatment group or the other. It's a high, and frequently unattainable, standard for quality initiatives. A 2003 tongue-in-cheek exploration of the limits of the randomized trial, published in the *British Medical Journal*, addressed the problem. A proper study of parachutes' effectiveness "in preventing major trauma related to gravitational challenge," the authors pointed out, would require that a random set of individuals jump from a height without parachutes. Our experience of life leads us to be confident about preferring parachutes to a free fall, but where's the proof?[23] To make this point even clearer, a 2018 study in the same journal randomized patients to jump out of airplanes with and without a parachute. The catch? The study was only able to recruit patients willing to jump without parachutes out of an airplane required that it be stationary and at ground level. The takeaway? Humans know better than to jump out of airplanes with backpacks on instead of parachutes![24]

There have been evidence-based studies showing that the longer a Foley remains in a patient, the greater the likelihood of infection. However, a randomized controlled trial of the CAUTI bundle would be difficult since it would require hospitals to withhold appropriate management from ill patients. Rather, the CAUTI prevention bladder bundle is a best practice approach, approved by the medical community as a whole. It is also a collection of items with a range of scientific support. There is stronger evidence for those items that speak directly to the Foley's length of stay in a patient, for instance, than for those that require aseptic insertion (as opposed to "clean" insertion). Several new external catheter options have been developed recently for women, and these devices appear logically to pose a lower risk of CAUTI[8] to the patient compared to an indwelling device, but we encourage hospitals to collect, share, and publish data from nurses and patients regarding the experience of using the devices. Other possible complications include skin breakdown related to contact with the wicking materials and suction or changes in nursing practice related to turning or skin care that could occur compared to standard care of a patient requiring skin care for incontinence without catheter use.

In the next chapter, we describe interventions for prevention of CLABSI, recognizing that the scientific evidence for CLABSI interventions has been considerably stronger than for CAUTI interventions, particularly as studies of CLABSI interventions have benefited from more rigorous randomized control trial designs than those of most CAUTI interventions.[15]

SUGGESTIONS FOR FURTHER READING

Gould CV, Umscheid CA, Agarwal RK, Kuntz G, Pegues DA, Healthcare Infection Control Practices Advisory Committee (HICPAC). Guideline for Prevention of catheter-associated urinary tract infections 2009. Infect Control Hosp Epidemiol 2010;31:319–326.

This guide both updates and expands the original CDC guidelines for prevention of catheter-associated urinary tract infections from 1981. This edition, often referred to as the "HICPAC Guidelines," provides examples of appropriate and inappropriate indications for indwelling urethral catheter use and was developed using a targeted, systematic review of the best available evidence, though their final indications were based primarily on expert consensus.

Lo E, Nicolle LE, Coffin SE, et al. Strategies to prevent catheter-associated urinary tract infections in acute care hospitals: 2014 update. Infect Control Hosp Epidemiol. 2014;35:464–479.

In this compendium, the authors highlighted some of the practical recommendations for acute care hospitals in their efforts to prevent CAUTI. Using the most up-to-date evidence and presented in a concise format, strategies for CAUTI detection, prevention, and performance measures are reviewed.

Meddings J, Saint S, Fowler KE, et al. The Ann Arbor Criteria for Appropriate Urinary Catheter Use in Hospitalized Medical Patients: Results Obtained by Using the RAND/ UCLA Appropriateness Method. Ann Intern Med. 2015;162:S1–S34.

As complications from indwelling Foley catheters have been increasingly recognized, this study sought to develop criteria for appropriate and inappropriate use of Foley catheters, as well as the use of three common alternatives to indwelling catheter use: intermittent straight catheters, external catheters, and noncatheter strategies for urine collection and skin protection. A multidisciplinary panel applied the RAND/UCLA Appropriateness Method to develop these criteria for hospitalized medical patients.

Meddings J, Skolarus TA, Fowler KE, et al. Michigan Appropriate Perioperative (MAP) criteria for urinary catheter use in common general and orthopaedic surgeries: results obtained using the RAND/UCLA Appropriateness Method. BMJ Qual Saf. 2019;28:56–66.

In this study, a multidisciplinary panel applied the RAND/UCLA Appropriateness Method to develop these criteria for appropriate perioperative use of indwelling urinary catheters for patients undergoing common general surgery procedures such as appendectomy, cholecystectomy, hernia repair, and colorectal procedures; and common orthopedic procedures such as elective knee arthroplasty, as well as hip arthroplasty and hip fracture repair.

Rotter ML. Semmelweis' sesquicentennial: a little-noted anniversary of handwashing. Curr Opin Infect Dis. 1998;11:457–460.

This review describes Hungarian obstetrician Ignaz Philipp Semmelweis's achievements from 150 years ago. In addition to documenting Semmelweis's observation of the importance of hand hygiene in disease prevention, Rotter discusses the current lack of compliance by some health professionals and concludes that 150 years later, hand hygiene "still remains an educational problem to be solved."

Types of Interventions

Central Line–Associated Bloodstream Infection

> So convenient a thing it is to be a reasonable creature, since it enables
> one to find or make a reason for every thing one has a mind to do.
>
> —Benjamin Franklin

At this very moment, a hospitalized patient somewhere in the world is undergoing the placement of a central venous catheter (CVC). Little do they or the operator performing the procedure know that this technique was first introduced in 1905 but almost never saw the light of day because the German inventor, Fritz Bleichröder, thought it had no practical value in 1905. Fortunately for us, Bleichröder changed his mind several years later, and central venous catheterization is now a cornerstone of modern medicine. Although central catheters vary in design, they have in common the fact that they are threaded into a vein (in either the trunk or the arm of the body) and are advanced until they terminate in a large vessel near the heart. CVCs provide reliable and dependable access to the deep venous system, carrying nutrients, medicines, or blood, and can remain in place for weeks on end.

For all of their blessings, these devices can be dangerous or even deadly. Clots may form around the catheter within the veins, setting in motion a coagulation cascade that may cause thrombosis or embolism. More pertinent to this chapter is the risk that bacterial pathogens will gain access to the bloodstream through the entry site of the device or from the catheter hub. Each year, these central line–associated bloodstream infections (CLABSIs) kill 12% to 25% of the more than 250,000 patients who develop them.[1]

By the turn of the century, researchers had developed effective methods to prevent CLABSI, but implementation of these evidence-based practices was slow. In 2004, the nonprofit Institute for Healthcare Improvement launched its nationwide 100,000 Lives Campaign, which included CLABSI prevention as a specific target. The results were impressive. Between 2001 and 2009, the rate of CLABSI in intensive care units (ICUs) was reduced by 58%, with substantial human and financial benefits. In 2009, compared to 2001, up to 6,000 fewer lives were lost to CLABSI, and medical costs were cut by $414 million.[2] This progress has continued, with recent point prevalence estimates showing continued reduction in the rates of CLABSI in 2018.[3]

In 2003, the Keystone Center of the Michigan Health and Hospital Association launched the Keystone ICU Initiative, which focused on implementing a bundle of evidence-based practices within a checklist to reduce CLABSI in more than 100 ICUs across the state of Michigan. This federally funded and evidence-based intervention focused on implementing a series of evidence-based steps each and every time a CVC was placed in a critical care setting. The intervention was a success and led to significantly reduced rates of CLABSI, from 7.7 infections at baseline to 1.4 infections 18 months later.[4] A similar intervention conducted at all 174 of the Veterans Health Administration's ICUs also succeeded in cutting CLABSI rates from 3.8 per 1,000 catheter days in 2006 to 1.8 per 1,000 days in 2009.[5]

The progress in CLABSI reduction has not come without new challenges. For example, early reductions in CLABSI rates were limited to the ICUs, as most CVCs were placed in this setting. Today, however, 70% of patients with central lines are located outside the ICU, and many of these lines are not clinically necessary;[6,7] therefore, the CLABSI incidence in these non-ICU units remains sizable, often rivaling or exceeding rates of CLABSI in

ICUs.[8] As a result, more and more hospitals are developing initiatives tailored to control CLABSI beyond the ICU.

The central line most used outside the ICU is called the peripherally inserted central catheter (PICC), which is inserted in the smaller, peripheral veins of the arm. First reported in 1972 by Dr. Verne Hoshal (a University of Michigan–trained surgeon), PICC use has grown tremendously over the past two decades. Because PICCs are placed in the veins of the arm under ultrasound guidance, they are relatively easier and safer to place than central lines in the veins of the neck and chest. Those advantages have multiplied with the proliferation of specialized vascular access teams, including qualified inserters. PICCs also offer a convenient and painless way for patients to receive treatments and undergo daily blood draws. The end result is that, far more than in the past, large numbers of sicker patients are being treated outside the ICU with PICCs, and many patients are sent home with the device in place to continue therapies such as antibiotics and chemotherapy outside the hospital.

For many years, there was little recognition of a trade-off between benefits and risks after PICC placement. While PICCs' lower rate of insertion complications was fueling its growth relative to central lines, the risk of downstream complications such as infection and thrombosis was little understood. And, it was not widely perceived that using a PICC in a patient who has difficult-to-access veins might not be the most judicious use of the device. These challenges came to the fore as PICCs began to be used widely. Reports of patient harm started to emerge. For example, a pediatric hospital reported that many of its patients had received PICCs for short time periods and had often undergone repeated placements that, on review, could have been avoided altogether. Another study found a high rate of adverse events, including blood clots and bloodstream infections—questioning whether the device should be used in all patients. But because most complications happened outside of ICU settings, developing a consistent evidence-based approach to synthesize the risks and benefits of PICCs remained challenging.

Research led by University of Michigan faculty and other scientists across the world has shed new light on these issues, leading to restraint in the use of these devices.[9] For example, meta-analyses have supported the belief that PICCs are associated with lower insertion complications than CVCs.[10] However, *major* complications such as infection occur just as commonly with PICCs in hospitalized and critically ill settings as with other central lines.[11,12] After all, there is nothing magical about a PICC when it comes to infection; just like traditional central lines, they are polyurethane catheters through which bacteria may gain entry into the bloodstream. Additional research showed that noninfectious complications—especially deep vein thrombosis—were actually more common with PICCs, with the greatest risk occurring in those patients who might benefit most from PICCs—those with cancer and in the intensive care setting.[1,13] The studies posed an important conundrum: Given these possible risks to patient safety, exactly when should PICCs be used? (See Appendix E.)

Efforts to answer that question led to a new concept: Central lines such as PICCs should be used only when necessary as a means to prevent catheter-associated harms. But how would a clinician know when a PICC or another central line was truly the best choice? The criteria generated for making that decision—the Michigan Appropriateness Guide for Intravenous Catheters (MAGIC), which is summarized in Appendix E (Appendix Figures E.1–E.4 and Box E.1)—focuses not only on PICCs, but also on six other commonly used peripheral and central venous access devices. After all, it is not enough to tell providers when they should versus should not use a PICC; they need guidance regarding what kind of device makes the most clinical sense. As a result of MAGIC, healthcare providers now have an evidence-based framework to use when making decisions about vascular access. The guidance within MAGIC also covers the intended duration of access and the nature of the proposed infusion.

MAGIC has been adopted by hundreds of hospitals in the United States and around the world. Reports from these centers indicate that its use not only has led to the selection of more appropriate devices, but also has reduced rates of complications.[14-16] Implementation of MAGIC using administrative data and electronic health records has made making the choice of the safest catheter easier for clinicians and healthcare providers.

   Though there has been much progress, some hospitals still report high
rates of CLABSI. There are several key reasons. The culture in the hospital may not hold CLABSI prevention important enough to pursue rig-
orously. Decisions about when to use a central line may not be occurring
in an evidence-based way. For example, even though criteria like MAGIC
provide guidance on when to use or not use a PICC, many subspecialists
such as oncologists or critical care physicians continue to choose them
over other devices based on convenience. The hospital's adherence to the
CLABSI bundle may not rise to the high level of commitment that is associated with significant improvement. To put it simply, many hospitals
want to see fewer infections but do not commit the resources in terms of
staff and time to ensure that audits, education, and troubleshooting are
being performed regularly. CLABSI rates may remain high in hospitals
that care for more complex patients. This is particularly true for larger academic medical centers that receive the sickest of the sick and have many
trainee physicians and nurses providing patient care. In fact, unlike catheter placement, the evidence for how best to maintain and care for vascular catheters is scant. This gap is important as insertion represents just
1% of the life of the catheter; how it is managed in the many days after-
ward often has much more to do with infection than whether the insertion
bundle was followed. And by the same token, the strategies for preventing
CLABSI outside the ICU are less defined than those for the ICU.
   As was the case in the catheter-associated urinary tract infection (CAUTI) prevention agenda, our model hospital's first step in
combatting CLABSI is to make sure that a vascular catheter is only
inserted if it is absolutely necessary. The Michigan Appropriateness
Guide for Intravenous Catheters helps in this decision-making as it
directs providers to less-invasive alternatives such as midlines and
ultrasound-guided peripheral intravenous access rather than central
access, if appropriate. The success of MAGIC has also led to a new mul-
tinational initiative focused on developing appropriateness criteria for
pediatric populations.[17] Dubbed "miniMAGIC," it indicates whether
use of a peripheral catheter or CVC is appropriate for ages neonate to
adolescent and echoes its older brother in focusing on evidence-based

recommendations and, wherever possible, calling for the use of the least invasive device to prevent harm.[17]

The model hospital recognizes that the longer any device such as a central line stays in place, the greater the risk of infection. As a result, the hospital's CLABSI prevention bundle emphasizes the need to remove the catheter as soon as possible. One means to that end is the iDECIDED tool.[18] iDECIDED offers a standardized, multidisciplinary way of assessing catheters daily to determine whether the catheter is functional and still clinically necessary, which is to say, still in the patient's best interest. The other evidence-based CLABSI bundle elements—initiated with the aid of a checklist (see Box 4.1)—at our model hospital.

- Hand hygiene: Use soap and water or an alcohol-based cleanser when preparing to insert a central line or when doing any maintenance care or lab draws from a central line.
- Use maximum sterile barriers during insertion, including face mask, gloves, hair covering, sterile gown, and full-body sterile drapes to cover the entire patient.
- Proper antiseptic: Use alcohol-containing chlorhexidine gluconate to clean the skin when the catheter is inserted.
- Preferred veins: Avoid the femoral vein when possible.
- Review each central line daily to determine whether it is still necessary based on appropriateness criteria[19]; promptly remove unnecessary devices.

At our model hospital, the chief medical officer, an intensivist herself, shows her support of the initiative by emphasizing the importance of using alcohol-containing chlorhexidine over povidone-iodine as a skin cleanser. In fact, she extended the use of chlorhexidine for skin antisepsis beyond line insertion to catheter maintenance by placing chlorhexidine-impregnated sponge dressings over the entry site of the catheters—now a Level 1 recommendation from the Centers for Disease Control and Prevention. As well, each morning during rounds in the ICU, she ensures there is a multidisciplinary discussion evaluating

Box 4.1

CENTRAL LINE INFECTION PREVENTION CHECKLIST

- Wash hands with soap before treating the patient.
- Clean the patient's skin with chlorohexidine antiseptic.
- Put sterile drapes over the entire patient.
- Wear a surgical mask, hat, sterile gown, and gloves while carrying out the line insertion.
- Put a sterile semitransparent dressing over the insertion site once the line is in.

Source: Developed by Pronovost and colleagues[4] and adapted from Gawande.[20]

the necessity of all the lines in the unit, including central lines. She implemented the iDECIDED tool[18,21] as the structure through which to have these conversations—thus creating a routine process that also documents these bedside discussions.

When a central line is being inserted at the model hospital, the hospital protocol empowers nurses to stop the procedure if the bundle guidelines are not being followed. When that happens, a secondary goal is to avoid confrontation between nurse and physician.

At one of the hospitals we visited, a resident physician routinely neglected to wear a hat when she inserted a central line. Finally, the nurse manager, holding a clipboard and pen, approached the doctor just before an insertion. "Let's see," the nurse said, "You're wearing a mask. OK. Good. Let's see, were you going to wear a hat?" When the resident challenged her, the nurse replied, "I'm filling out this form for Dr. [Name of senior physician omitted]." "Wha . . . wha . . . Okay, gimme a hat," the resident said.

Leaders at the model hospital recognized that the care and maintenance of devices was highly variable. To standardize the approach, the chief medical officer worked with the leads of infection control and nursing to create a standardized catheter care kit. This kit includes all of the necessary materials needed for catheter maintenance—sterile gloves, prefilled saline syringes for flushing, a small sterile drape to place around the catheter, semitransparent dressings, and the chlorhexidine patch—in a small package with a graphical illustration of the steps to provide care. Having all the materials needed for catheter care in one place and consistently available regardless of whether the patient is in an ICU or a ward setting greatly improved the consistency of care and maintenance. The kit became so popular in the hospital that, with the aid of a manufacturer, it was commercially marketed.

An infection preventionist at a hospital that adopted a similar approach told us about its impact: "It's becoming more and more difficult to not use [chlorhexidine rather than betadine] because that's what's available. People still have their stashes, it's a big hospital, but it's harder and harder."

NEW APPROACHES TO CLABSI PREVENTION

The States Targeting Reduction in Infections Via Engagement (STRIVE)[22] initiative described in Chapter 3 also included a two-tier approach for prioritizing CLABSI interventions (Appendix C, Figure C.2)[23] based on a systematic literature review[24] and expert experience, and it included a CLABSI Guide to Patient Safety (GPS) (Appendix D, Box D.2)[25] online assessment tool. Tier 1 of the CLABSI modules in STRIVE matched up with the practices of our model hospital, reviewed above, from avoiding the femoral site for CVC insertion to the removal of the CVC as soon as it is no longer clinically necessary.

The Tier 2 CLABSI prevention effort (Appendix C, Figure C.2), like that for CAUTI, included a list of enhanced practices, requiring a greater expenditure of human and material resources than those in Tier 1. Participants filled out a CLABSI GPS, modeled after the validated CAUTI GPS.[25] It consisted of a self-administered series of yes/no questions designed to pinpoint the particular difficulties a hospital was having with its CLABSI intervention. The answers then triggered a series of targeted solutions the hospital could pursue.

For example, when a hospital's responses indicated that providers were having difficulty placing the appropriate catheter or with the prompt removal of central lines when they were no longer needed, Tier 2 advised the hospital to implement multidisciplinary CLABSI rounds to cope with both problems. It suggested that the rounds be headed by a lead member of the intervention team, such as the critical care fellow, ICU attending physician, or charge nurse. The hospital was also urged to adopt standardized line audit checklists (such as iDECIDED[18]) as a way to achieve early CVC removal.

Studies have shown that high-performing CLABSI prevention units are often aware of CLABSI rates in their hospital and share a sense of pride or disappointment when rates improve or drop. Tier 2 recommended making CLABSI-specific metrics available to front-line staff as a way to foster lagging teamwork during an intervention. In addition to prominent displays of the metrics, Tier 2 suggested giving such feedback on an individual, confidential level to increase nurses' cooperation—especially if there were outliers to the prevailing practice.

Any indication that a hospital was having problems with its CVC insertion and maintenance procedures inspired a Tier 2 response advising the hospital to undertake closer monitoring of those procedures. One approach was to assign a nurse to the task. An educational intervention was also proposed. A simulation-based program, for example, has been shown to increase ICU nurses' competency in catheter maintenance practices.

When a hospital's CLABSI rates remained high, notwithstanding its application of those earlier recommendations, Tier 2 suggests that the hospital consider using advanced, admittedly expensive, technologies. Antimicrobial-coated or -impregnated CVCs were among those listed, even though some recent trials of the devices have failed to provide definitive proof of their effectiveness in the setting of high infection rates. However, there is some evidence that antimicrobial PICCs can help with such high-risk groups as oncology patients and those on burn units. Other potential technologies listed included antithrombotic catheters and such novel materials as antiseptic-impregnated dressings. Some strategies STRIVE recommended to reduce CLABSI rates over time included investments in building a vascular access team that was skilled in peripheral access, the use of ultrasound, and managing patients with difficult venous access.

Tier 2's final and most drastic suggestion was a root cause analysis of each of a hospital's CLABSI cases. That would call for the hospital to identify and clearly describe the problem; create a timeline from a patient's baseline normal to the moment the infection was diagnosed; and separate the root cause from other causal factors. The results can reveal lapses in safety, key themes associated with adverse events, and foster communication among intervention team members.

A study[26] of the STRIVE intervention found that it did not yield a substantial overall reduction of CLABSI rates or rates of central line use at the 337 hospitals that reported outcome data. All was not lost, however, as there were significant reductions in some hospitals—including a 50% cutback in 50 participating institutions. Importantly, only 63% of the hospitals actually focused on CLABSI reduction as a priority, perhaps blunting the overall effectiveness of the intervention when examining all hospitals as a whole. The elements within STRIVE, after all, were all based on evidence suggesting benefit; what often was missing is how well the elements were implemented.

The results of the STRIVE project, the study[26] concluded, is that a one-size-fits-all approach to CLABSI prevention in high-rate hospitals may not be the most effective. For some higher performing hospitals, strategies such as education and an outside, guided implementation may work well. Conversely, lower performing institutions may not see benefits from this approach because they do not have the right people in place to lead or lack the structure through which to implement recommendations. They may require a more activist, boots-on-the-ground approach. The study noted that a strategy with both external and internal components had been used successfully in a Veterans Affairs setting when sites struggled to implement a primary care model. Perhaps this hybrid approach, which brought both evidence and human capital to the table, could help hospitals struggling to prevent CLABSI.

SUGGESTIONS FOR FURTHER READING

Chopra V, Flanders SA, Saint S, et al. The Michigan Appropriateness Guide for Intravenous Catheters (MAGIC): Results from a Multispecialty Panel Using the RAND/UCLA Appropriateness Method. Ann Intern Med. 2015;163:S1–S40.

   As PICC use has grown substantially, this study sought to develop criteria for appropriate and inappropriate PICC use based on patient population, indication for insertion, and duration of use. An international, multidisciplinary panel applied the RAND/UCLA Appropriateness Method to develop these criteria.

Gawande A. The checklist: if something so simple can transform intensive care, what else can it do? New Yorker. 2007, December 3:86–101.

   In his engaging and thought-provoking style, Gawande discusses the modern challenges facing ICUs and their staff. Using the work of Peter Pronovost, MD, PhD, and the successful results of the central line checklist he implemented first at Johns Hopkins Hospital and later throughout the state of Michigan, Gawande explores the complexity of caring for the sickest patients given the multitude of opportunities to introduce error.

Marschall J, Mermel LA, Fakih M, et al. Strategies to prevent central line-associated bloodstream infections in acute care hospitals: 2014 update. Infect Control Hosp Epidemiol. 2014;35:753–771.

   As with the catheter-associated urinary tract infection compendium, the authors updated the previously published guidelines for CLABSI prevention in acute care hospitals. Using the most up-to-date evidence and presented in a concise format, strategies for CLABSI detection, prevention, and performance measures are reviewed.

Moureau N, Chopra V. Indications for peripheral, midline and central catheters: summary of the MAGIC recommendations. Br J Nurs. 2016;25:S15–S24.

   This article summarizes the work and recommendations of the panel that developed the Michigan Appropriateness Guide for Intravenous Catheters (MAGIC). Selection of the most appropriate vascular access device is often complicated by patient factors such as difficult intravenous access as well as obesity, diabetes, and other chronic conditions. These criteria guide clinicians toward the most appropriate device—a necessity in order to avoid potentially serious complications.

O'Grady NP, Alexander M, Burns LA, et al. Summary of recommendations: guidelines for the prevention of intravascular catheter-related infections. Clin Infect Dis. 2011;52:1087–1099.

   This report, prepared by a multidisciplinary working group in collaboration with more than 15 professional societies, replaces the 2002 Guideline for Prevention of Intravascular Catheter-Related Infections. Each of the recommendations is categorized based on the strength of existing scientific data, theoretical rationale, applicability, and economic impact.

Swaminathan L, Flanders S, Rogers M, et al. Improving PICC use and outcomes in hospitalised patients: an interrupted time series study using MAGIC criteria. BMJ Qual Saf. 2018;27:271–278.

This study sought to understand whether the use of MAGIC could reduce inappropriate PICC use. This quasi-experimental, interrupted time series study compared implementation of MAGIC at one hospital versus nine control hospitals that did not follow the guide. This quality improvement project showed that implementation of MAGIC modestly improved PICC use appropriateness and reduced complications associated with the use of these devices compared to the control hospitals, which saw no significant changes.

Building the Team

Never doubt that a small group of thoughtful, concerned citizens can change the world. Indeed it is the only thing that ever has.

—MARGARET MEAD

"Surgeons are very tribal," the chief of staff said, discussing the difficulty that an infection prevention leader might have trying to bring his message to a group of surgeons. "The first thing we're going to do is we're going to say, 'Look, you're not one of us.' The way to get buy-in from surgeons is you got to have a surgeon on your team."

In this chapter, we move from specific devices and technical practices of infection prevention to focus on the adaptive side—the people side. We return to the model hospital to see how our catheter-associated urinary tract infection (CAUTI) project manager goes about selecting her team—and how they prepare for the all-important task of implementation. Their ability to predict and find solutions for the personal and institutional roadblocks ahead will decide the fate of the initiative. This chapter uses CAUTI as the example infection for identifying common challenges to implementation and key adaptive strategies to meet those challenges, with many parallels to best practices seen in central line–associated bloodstream infection (CLABSI) prevention teams.

A successful infection prevention initiative requires, above all, highly motivated and effective team members and a maximum of forward planning. The project manager, the nurse and physician champions, and any other team members need to think long and hard about the problems they are likely to face in pursuing the initiative. They need to search, ahead of time, for ways to confront or avoid those problems, such as making sure there is a surgeon on the team.

The team's primary goal is to create what is, in effect, a "people bundle," the social and adaptive counterpart to the technical focus of the bladder bundle. Too often, in the effort to effect change and implement best practices, short shrift is given to the "people" aspect of the process. It takes a village—the widespread cooperation of a hospital's nurses and doctors— to secure a successful quality initiative. And it takes an organized, intensive team effort, implementing a people bundle, to gain that cooperation.

At our model hospital, building a team is the new project manager's first order of business. Why the team approach? Why not just a letter from the hospital's chief executive officer or chief medical officer announcing a new safety initiative? Maybe something along these lines: "From this day forward, all bedside nurses will fill out a checklist at shift's end reporting on the presence of Foleys in their units and will ask physicians to remove unnecessary catheters." Because it doesn't work. In fact, a top-down approach can often have the reverse result. Note the effect of hospitals' continuing insistence that all their healthcare workers must have a yearly flu vaccination: a nationwide response rate of just 67% for the 2011–2012 season.[1] It takes more than a C-suite command to convince bedside nurses to adopt an operational change that will add to their already substantial workload.

In this chapter, we describe the team recruiting process for a medical floor–based intervention at the midsize, 250-bed model hospital. The personnel and structure of a team will generally vary with the size of the facility. At a small hospital, the team might consist of just the project manager and a nurse champion since the number of patients with indwelling urinary catheters is typically no more than a handful. A large hospital might have a process improvement team already in place and ready to take on any safety initiative. The creation of a project team will also vary somewhat depending on what part of the hospital is to be targeted—the medical floor, as here, or the operating room or emergency department (ED), where the vast majority of Foleys are inserted. (More on that topic is discussed further in the chapter.)

RECRUITING A NURSE CHAMPION

The nurse champion at our model hospital will most likely be a nurse unit manager, a charge nurse, a nurse educator, or a staff nurse. Nurse champions need to know their way around the hospital hierarchy but be independent minded in terms of finding solutions. They should have a strong commitment to patient safety, and they must be on good terms with their colleagues. By way of contrast, when a nurse executive or director of nursing becomes nurse champion, there is the danger that the bedside nurses will view the infection prevention initiative as just another occasion for obeying the boss, rather than as a nurse-based effort to better serve patients. Far more than the physician champion, the nurse champion will be the embodiment of the project to the people who will decide its fate, the bedside nurses. The right nurse champion will have the strongest insight and ideas for how to convince bedside nurses to do something that may improve patient safety while also minimizing the negative impacts on the nurses, such as the extra bedside effort required.

Given the right set of circumstances, a bedside nurse can be a formidable champion for infection prevention initiatives. We know of one example of that arrangement—a bedside nurse who attended planning meetings as well as the monthly meetings postimplementation on their personal time, and whose dedication to infection prevention became, well, contagious among nursing colleagues throughout the hospital.

The nurse champion will, inevitably, be a busy person. To win the nurse's participation, the project manager at the model hospital begins by promising that the nurse will be given time off from clinical duties to attend planning and reporting sessions and ensuring that other project duties will be able to be handled during regular shifts. The manager makes it clear that the nurse champion will be a full partner in the infection prevention enterprise and that the project will have the full support of the hospital leadership and other staff members. High on the support list will be the case managers, who equate reduced complications with lower costs and who understand that the early removal of a catheter can reduce a patient's length of stay. Infection preventionists will also be in the champion's corner not only because the bladder bundle can reduce urinary tract infection, but also because it can cut back on antimicrobial use.

The project manager lets the potential nurse champion know that his or her work will be recognized in annual evaluation appraisals and in communications with the chief nursing officer. Other possible public acknowledgments could be an article in the hospital newsletter or a "nurse champion award" presented during a hospital town hall meeting or other staff recognition event. Above all, the manager appeals to the nurse's concern for the comfort and safety of patients—the concern that inspired his or her career to begin with and is the primary force behind the intervention.

ENLISTING A PHYSICIAN CHAMPION

To enlist a physician champion, the project manager should look among the hospital epidemiologists, hospitalists, infectious diseases specialists, and those whose specialty is relevant to the particular infection prevention target, urologists in this case. The project manager wants a physician who has pride in the hospital's culture of excellence or concern over the lack of one. The project manager also seeks a person who has the ear of the hospital administration and the respect of his or her peers, a doctors' doctor, and someone who has the patience to hear out people who disagree with his or her point of view. The search for volunteers is complicated by the fact that some of the doctors are not employees of the hospital. As private practitioners, they may lack a sense of identification with the facility, and they are comparatively free of its authority. Convincing any physician, employee, or nonemployee to take on extra work beyond their current practice is likely to be a tough assignment.

Some hospitals have experimented with giving employee physicians a financial bonus to shoulder quality improvement roles, but, as one medical director told us, that's "kind of a slippery slope." Paying doctors to take part in a patient-centered intervention seems inappropriate to us. We see no problem, though, with temporarily relieving the physician of some of his or her responsibilities or, as was done in one hospital, recognizing a member of the medical staff with a "physician champion" award, complete with a certificate signed by the hospital's chief of staff and a gift certificate to a local restaurant.

In her discussions with potential physician champions, the project manager at the model hospital emphasizes the need to take action against infection in general and in this hospital in particular. She emphasizes that the project's protocols are reliable, are straight from the Centers for Disease Control and Prevention (CDC), and offers examples of successful infection prevention interventions in nearby facilities. She informs the potential champion that the hospital administration has given the project a high priority, and that she and the administration view doctors as full partners in the project, not as barriers. She cites the medical reasons why physician champions can count on the support of their colleagues (e.g., rehabilitation specialists and geriatricians because Foleys reduce patient mobility and urologists because the insertion and removal of the devices can lead to urethral damage and other patient-related injuries). Early and often, she assures the potential champion that the champion role will not take too much time. They will not, for instance, be expected to attend all meetings or be otherwise involved in matters unrelated to clinical concerns, such as budget discussions or internal promotion plans or working out details of data collection. The chief responsibility will be to share the details of the intervention with colleagues and gain their cooperation.

In making her team selections, the project manager needs to avoid choosing people on the basis of their job title. Unfortunately, titles don't guarantee that a person will be appropriate for this task. As a case in point, for an intervention to prevent healthcare-associated infection (HAI), the infection preventionist might seem like an obvious choice for project manager. And we have, indeed, encountered some infection preventionists who were perfect for this task because they were on cordial terms with everyone in their hospitals, doctors and nurses alike; cared deeply about the intervention; and knew just what buttons to push to keep a project on track. But we also found others who were fixated on surveillance and infection rates and were not well versed in the behavioral changes necessary to ensure a successful intervention.

Hospitalists are also seemingly natural members or leaders of the project team. These physicians, who now number approximately 60,000 in the United States alone, spend their days interacting with nurses and patients. They tend to be considerably younger than most other physicians in the hospital and to have more of a team-centered approach to medicine and thus may have far better relationships with nurses. But because their age could be a handicap in dealing with older doctors, hospitalists may sometimes not be ideal for leadership roles in an intervention.

The project manager also needs to beware of the tendency to choose from the same pool of people who always seem to get tapped to lead quality improvement projects. They often end up being overcommitted and unable to devote the necessary time and energy to a given initiative.

Aside from the project manager and the nurse and physician champions, the team will generally include someone to handle data, typically an infection preventionist or a member of the quality improvement department. He or she will collate information—specifically, the presence of a Foley, the explanation for its original insertion or continued use, and any indication of a healthcare-associated urinary tract infection—and feed it back to the floor unit involved and to the hospital office responsible for sending the results to the CDC. (See Figure 5.1, an example of a urinary catheter data collection sheet.) In order to bring in people who will be close to the action, the addition of other team members may be delayed until after the team has selected the medical unit that will be the campaign's first target.

The executive sponsor, the head of nursing, is an ex officio member of the team, who sits down with the project manager every two weeks to monitor the intervention's progress, and makes an occasional, unannounced appearance at meetings. The sponsor expects that the project manager will clear major decisions with her. She wants the team as a

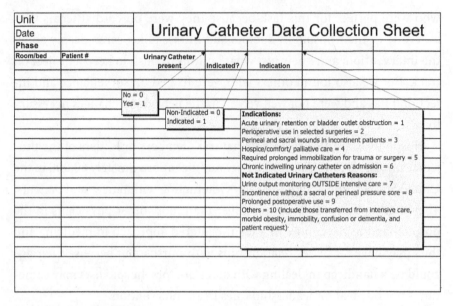

Figure 5.1 Example of a urinary catheter data collection sheet.

whole to understand that she represents the hospital leadership's continuing interest in the initiative, and that she is there for them if a need arises, although, she also makes clear, she has every confidence that they will handle this assignment on their own with flying colors (see Table 5.1).

HOW THE TEAM OPERATES

In a quality improvement initiative, as in so many of life's endeavors, nothing succeeds like success. For the team at the model hospital to convince administrators and medical leaders that the infection prevention intervention is effective and worth introducing throughout the institution, clear proof will be required. This is how the team plans to go about it.

The intervention will start small, with a single 20-bed unit, so that team members can easily monitor results and quickly resolve any problems that crop up during the implementation. The project manager is looking for a unit that has a track record of cooperating with earlier quality initiatives—there's no need to look for trouble—but is not in the midst of too many

Table 5.1 An Example of the Roles and Responsibilities of the Members of a Team[a]

Role or Responsibility	Example of Personnel to Consider and Some Advice
Project coordinator/ team manager	Infection preventionist, quality manager, nurse manager *When selecting a team leader, consider whether the team leader has successfully led another quality improvement project. Generally, the leadership skills and previous success are more important than the job title or content expertise.*
Nurse champion	Nurse manager, charge nurse, staff nurse, nurse educator *For a CAUTI prevention initiative, if you do not already have a nurse champion, consider a charge nurse or nurse manager rather than a bedside nurse. The charge nurse or nurse manager generally has more time away from the bedside and is thus able to help with other initiatives. In addition, these nurses generally have more influence over other nurses. This person is needed to obtain buy-in from other nurses because often these CAUTI initiatives can involve additional nursing effort (monitoring indwelling urinary catheter placement, monitoring indications, spending more time toileting patients, and possibly involving data collection).*
Physician champion	Hospitalist, hospital epidemiologist, infectious diseases specialist, geriatrician, emergency physician, urologist *A physician champion can be key to the success of the initiative. Try to involve a physician who is highly regarded or has the ear of other physicians. If you do not have access to a physician who is willing to be an actively involved physician champion, then consider selecting a respected physician who is willing to lend his or her name to this initiative without doing most of the actual work.*
Data collection, monitoring, and reporting	Infection preventionist, quality manager, patient safety officer *For a CAUTI prevention initiative, someone must be responsible for collecting data on CAUTI outcomes and indwelling urinary catheter prevalence. This can be the same person who currently collects these data for the hospital.*

[a] Adapted from Fakih et al.[2]

initiatives at the moment. The unit should also have a full share of Foleys in place, as well as a high rate of CAUTI, so that the campaign improvement will be as impressive as possible.

After consulting with nursing staff familiar with the individual medical floor units, the team will choose three or four such units. The project manager will then arrange for the collection of key data from each of those units over a five-day period: the presence of a Foley, the explanation for its original insertion, and why it is currently still in place. In addition, information about the CAUTI rates in the units will be obtained from the infection preventionist. It is hoped that these baseline data will, when compared to data collected during and after implementation of the initiative, provide the proof needed to convince administration and clinical leaders to expand the campaign to other parts of the hospital. It will also determine which of the several units under consideration is best suited to be the campaign's first target.

The First Meeting

To open the first formal meeting of the team, which may also be attended by other interested hospital personnel, the project manager presents a larger vision of the intervention. Hospital infections are a national problem, she says, and it's a serious problem in this hospital; the chief executive officer is very concerned. Then the project manager switches gears and speaks of the needless human pain caused by CAUTI. She tells stories of actual patients at the hospital who developed a CAUTI and the suffering they endured, as well as the noninfectious complications that accompany use of the Foley. Her message is that this project is not simply another bureaucratic exercise, and it is not simply another research project dreamed up by academics; it is crucially important for the hospital and for its patients.

At the meeting, the project manager shares information from the published literature about what others have done to reduce the incidence of CAUTI and shows a video describing the components of the bladder bundle. The nurse champion answers any clinical questions attendees may have about the actual insertion and removal of the Foley as currently practiced in the hospital and explains the various alternatives to the indwelling catheter. The project manager then walks her listeners through the plans for the implementation process, rehearsing the various steps along the way, including her determination not to start the intervention during the summer vacation season. She solicits suggestions and clarifications.

An infection preventionist asks whether a computer-based self-learning module has been considered as a way to educate bedside nurses and physicians in the details of the bladder bundle. She says one had been used to good effect at the hospital where she had previously worked. The module explained the connection between Foleys and CAUTI and included directions for the proper placement and maintenance of the catheters. Those assigned to use the module were given a date for completion after which their understanding of the material was evaluated. The one thing the module lacked, she says, was sufficient emphasis on communicating the requirements of the bladder bundle to physicians. The project manager says that a self-learning module might be a good possibility if the intervention extends to the whole hospital.

The project manager is reminded of another computer-based, interactive program, this one developed by the US Department of Health and Human Services. It presents dramatized scenarios related to HAI prevention and gives clinicians a chance to "play it out before you live it out." The problem, she points out, is that the program is focused on other infections, not CAUTI.[3]

A nurse supervisor recalls encountering a real-life version of the agency's approach at a meeting devoted to improving nurse–physician relations. The nurses and doctors at the session took turns going through likely scenarios—a physician giving an inappropriate order for a Foley, for example, or a nurse asking a physician for an order to remove a catheter from a patient.

The project manager has finished drafting a new version of the hospital's CAUTI prevention policy and procedures to reflect the components of the bladder bundle. At the meeting, she passes around a copy of the draft, seeking feedback from the other team members. A nurse suggests that the draft should include having a nurse who is trained in the new catheter policy take part in daily rounds. That sets off a lively debate, which the project manager finally cuts off, pleading time pressures. She says she will raise the possibility verbally when she submits her draft to the project's executive sponsor but cautions that the leadership is unlikely to be ready to take that step.

She then outlines her plans for promoting the intervention within the hospital, building hospital-wide support for the day when the campaign spreads to other units, including the ED and intensive care units (ICUs). Educational posters will be hung in high-traffic spots such as nursing lounges and restrooms, and flyers will be distributed, proclaiming, "Get That Urinary Catheter Out!" and "Ex-Foley-Ate." Space will be set aside on the hospital's website and in its newsletters for a description of HAI and an announcement of the new initiative to deal with it. Campaign messages will also be regularly broadcast on social networks such as Facebook and Twitter.

But the most important promotion, the project manager insists, is the one that team members and their supporters will undertake in their daily contacts with hospital staff: the physicians in their conversations with colleagues and in presentations at grand rounds or at medical staff conferences; the nurses at morning report, at in-service training, and in one-on-one talks. To put a human face on the campaign, she urges them to use, where feasible, their own version of the emotional appeal with which she started the meeting. Convincing nurses and doctors to revise long-time routine procedures and winning their acceptance of a change in the nurse–doctor relationship along the way—all that, the project manager admits, is a tall order. It will take all of the team's persuasive powers, she warns, and that process should start as soon as possible.

The project manager also reports that three units have been chosen as potential candidates to be the initial target of the initiative. She says she has initiated the collection of baseline data from these units, and she promises to identify the ultimate target unit at the next meeting.

The Follow-Up

Ten days later, the project manager is as good as her word: She starts the follow-up meeting by announcing that the initiative will focus first on 4 West, a 20-bed unit with the best combination of willing nurses and indwelling urinary catheters. The nurse champion is already bringing the unit's nurse educator up to speed on the bladder bundle to help prepare her for her sessions explaining the intervention to the unit's bedside nurses. The rest of the meeting is devoted to rehearsing the implementation of the bladder bundle, making sure there is a standard operating procedure in place, and discussing potential problems. Does the unit have enough intermittent straight catheters on hand? Is there a portable bladder scanner on the unit? Are there other quality improvement activities underway or scheduled on 4 West that need to be coordinated with? Are there personal traits or quirks of the 4 West leadership that the team needs to watch out for? Will the nursing staff get with the program? Have the elements of the bundle been properly integrated into the patient record system?

The start of the implementation is scheduled for the following Monday. On Sunday, both the day and night nursing staffs receive text messages reminding them of the event. But there is no celebration—no ribbon cutting, no bagels—on Monday morning. This is not the first quality improvement program the unit has undertaken, and it will not be the last, and the staff has other fish to fry—catching up on weekend developments, for example.

But the executive sponsor does show up at the unit's morning meeting to emphasize the importance of the intervention. The nurse champion is there as well and will visit the unit most days during initial implementation, checking in with the unit manager and chatting with one or another of the nurses to see how the project is going. But it will be the task of the unit manager and the charge nurse to make sure the bedside nurses understand and are performing their key role in the project.

At least once a day, the nurses of 4 West are to become the "Foley police," or "catheter patrol," as many hospitals have dubbed them. They note on the Foley template on the computerized patient record system whether their patients have an indwelling catheter; if the device is newly inserted, the reason for its placement, and the reason that it is still in place. And, if there is not an appropriate reason for the catheter according to the bladder bundle, the nurses are to inform the physician and suggest the removal of the Foley. That's the theory, but as will be seen in Chapter 6, there can be a formidable chasm between theory and practice.

If the intervention succeeds on 4 West, if the use of Foleys decreases substantially and the infection rate drops, the campaign is scheduled to move on to other units and, eventually, to the ED and ICUs. The challenges will be substantial on the wards since each unit has its own personality and its variety of personalities, but the basic mode of operation is similar from one unit to the next. The ED and ICUs represent very different environments, compared to the medical floor and to each other. So as the campaign expands, the personnel of the project team will inevitably need to change to match the new target sites.

PREVENTING CAUTI IN THE EMERGENCY DEPARTMENT

The key to a successful CAUTI prevention initiative in an ED is the active participation of one or more emergency medicine physicians.[4] In that hectic and unpredictable environment, the physicians and nurses properly see themselves as serving on the front lines. As an ED chief put it, "When you are working in the pit, and see it the way we do, having one of us carry the ball brings a level of credibility to the table that outside physicians don't exactly bring." Nurses and doctors are more concerned about whether their patients are still breathing than about whether they have a catheter. It takes a member of the team to convince the ED that catheters count.

Traditionally, indwelling catheters have been placed automatically in ED patients with severe enough problems to require them to stay on in the hospital, and the nurses don't want them walking around. When the patients are ready to leave for the wards, the nurses seldom pause to remove the Foleys, which explains why most indwelling catheters on the medical wards come from the ED.

The first goal of the bladder bundle's project manager in the ED is to convince physicians and nurses to make sure a patient's condition warrants an indwelling catheter and to consider safer alternatives, such as a condom catheter or a bladder scanner with intermittent straight catheterization. The second goal is to convince them to have the Foleys removed, where appropriate, before the patients move to the medical floor. (At some hospitals, ED nurses said they left in catheters as a favor to the floor nurses, to save them the trouble of reinserting.)

The project leader can demonstrate the importance of the intervention by sharing with her team the latest data from the medical floor, particularly figures showing how many of the floor's Foleys started out in the ED and what percentage of them led to an infection. The project leader can call a meeting of physicians to seek their cooperation in the initiative. The most effective approach, though, is for the project leader and/or the nurse champion to spend a part of each day walking through the department, reminding everyone they see about the intervention, asking a nurse or a physician whether that Foley they are about to insert is really necessary, whether it meets the appropriateness criteria, or asking whether the patient being rolled toward the entrance to the wards has a Foley in place and whether it's still needed. "It took a while," one ED chief said, "but eventually they got the message, and they did not want to see us anymore. They knew their old habits were probably not best for the patient."

Research supports the potential for reducing catheter use by focusing on the ED. In a systems-based collaborative, the development and implementation of institutional guidelines for appropriate urinary catheter use in combination with the identification of clinical champions to promote adherence to the guidelines has successfully achieved statistically significant and sustained reductions in unnecessary urinary catheter placement in an ED intervention. Impressive results were recently demonstrated in a systems-based collaborative, though not in a state-based collaborative with hospitals from many systems.[5]

PREVENTING CAUTI IN THE INTENSIVE CARE UNIT

The ICU has its own team spirit, rooted in a feeling that it is a special place—the life-saving arm of the hospital—and it takes a team member to lead a successful initiative there. Project managers have their work cut out for them: As in the ED, the default position is to insert Foleys. In a unit whose nurses spend their days monitoring patients' symptoms on a maze of machines, interrupted by intermittent crises, the indwelling urinary catheter offers a touch of simplicity, an easy way to keep track of a patient's urinary output, especially in the case of seriously ill patients who need their output monitored by the hour. These patients will receive medications and fluids based on urine output measurements. But for many other critical care patients, especially those from the operating room, the immediate goal is to get them up and walking as soon as possible and having a Foley can delay that result.

Patients' stay in the ED is measured in hours, whereas intensive care patients typically spend several days there. That greatly increases the odds that a Foley, whether appropriately or inappropriately inserted, will have outlived its time and should be removed. Project managers need to see that "presence/rationale for Foley" is added to the daily checklists used by the ICU teams. However, it is important to recognize that some CAUTI interventions that have been quite successful in other environments—including other units of the hospital and in interventions in smaller collaboratives of hospitals—have not been successful in the ICU environment in recent collaboratives.[6-8] By way of contrast, there has been a stronger history of significant and sustained reductions in CLABSI in the ICU setting.[9-11]

PREVENTING CAUTI FOR THE POSTOPERATIVE PATIENT

Bladder bundle interventions have generally not devoted much time and energy to converting operating room personnel. When a surgery is going to run on for six hours or so, the indwelling catheter is a logical option. Shorter procedures are questionable in that regard, but many surgical personnel automatically and insistently use Foleys. Project managers should still consider getting buy-in from surgeons to add "discontinue Foley" to the postoperative order sets but need to be prepared for this not being warmly received by some surgical teams.

For example, we were told of an elective orthopedic procedure that was scheduled to last two hours. When a nurse prepared to insert a Foley, an observer familiar with the bladder bundle philosophy suggested that the catheter was not necessary based on the Michigan Appropriate Perioperative Criteria,[12] which include guidance regarding when it is safe to avoid placement of catheters (e.g., procedures like routine appendectomy, laparoscopic cholecystectomy, and unilateral elective knee or hip arthroplasty); when it is safe to use catheters but to remove them in the operating room before transfer to a postanesthesia unit or ward (e.g., hip arthroplasty for fracture, routine hemicolectomy); and procedures when postoperative catheter use is appropriate for one to four days depending on the complexity of the procedure and potential for pelvic nerve disruption (e.g., laparoscopic perineal resection). The anesthesiologist protested. He wanted that Foley, he said, because he didn't want to have to worry about urinary retention—he had enough other things to think about. He did not welcome the suggestion that CAUTI was also worth worrying about in the operating room. In such circumstances when clinicians of a particular discipline disagree with the literature supporting changes in practice, it can be helpful to employ leaders from within that same discipline to encourage practice change among their colleagues.

In the next chapter, we discuss the role of quality improvement leadership in the C-suite and among project managers and team champions. Topics include the varieties of leadership approaches and the power of emotional intelligence.

SUGGESTED FURTHER READING

Collins J. Good to Great and the Social Sectors. New York, NY: Harper Business; 2011.
Setting out to answer the question, "Can a good company become great?" this book looks in depth at 11 companies that made substantial improvements in their performance over time to see if there were any common traits among them. What the author discovered challenged much of the conventional wisdom of the time.

Damschroder LJ, Banaszak-Holl J, Kowalski CP, Forman J, Saint S, Krein SL. The role of the "champion" in infection prevention: results from a multisite qualitative study. Qual Saf Health Care. 2009;18:434–440.

In this multisite, mixed-methods study of 86 individuals at 14 VA and non-VA hospitals, Damschroder and colleagues looked at champions who led efforts to implement best practices to prevent HAI. Their findings suggest that the factors that influence the choice of champions vary with the type of practice implemented (new technology vs. behavioral changes), and that the quality of the organizational networks affects the effectiveness of the champions.

Dixon-Woods M, Bosk CL, Aveling EL, Goeschel CA, Pronovost PJ. Explaining Michigan: developing an ex post theory of a quality improvement program. Milbank Q. 2011;89:167–205.

The authors proposed an approach for developing ex post theories of interventional programs to better understand why and how programs work, using the example of the successful Michigan Keystone Project to Reduce Central Venous Catheter Bloodstream Infections in Intensive Care Units.

Fakih MG, Pena ME, Shemes S, et al. Effect of establishing guidelines on appropriate urinary catheter placement. Acad Emerg Med. 2010;17:337–340.

In this study, the authors sought to evaluate the effect of establishing institutional guidelines for appropriate urinary catheter placement and physician education in the ED of their academic medical center. They found that 15% of the patients had urinary catheters placed, but only 47% of those insertions had a documented physician's order. Among the documented, 75.5% of the catheters were appropriately indicated, compared to 52% when no such documentation was present. These results indicate that establishing guidelines for urinary catheter placement and physician education in the ED was associated with a marked reduction in utilization.

Greene MT, Fakih MG, Watson SR, Ratz D, Saint S. Reducing inappropriate urinary catheter use in the emergency department: comparing two collaborative structures. Infect Control Hosp Epidemiol. 2018;39:77–84.

In this study comparing the success of interventions to reduce urinary catheter use in a systems-based collaborative compared to a state-based collaborative, the systems-based collaborative achieved a statistically significant and sustained reduction in inappropriate urinary catheter use by implementation of an ED-focused intervention that included institutional guidelines and clinical champions.

Patel PK, Gupta A, Vaughn VM, Mann JD, Ameling JM, Meddings J. Review of strategies to reduce central line–associated bloodstream infection (CLABSI) and catheter-associated urinary tract infection (CAUTI) in adult ICUs. J Hosp Med. 2018;13:105–116.

This systematic review compared and summarized the broad published literature describing the impact of interventions for reducing CLABSI and CAUTI in the intensive care setting and categorized these interventions in a conceptual model of targets for prioritization to disrupt the life cycle of vascular or urinary catheters: avoidance of unnecessary catheters, ensuring aseptic insertion, optimizing maintenance care, and prompting removal when the catheters are no longer clinically necessary.

The Importance of Leadership and Followership

My own definition of leadership is this: The capacity and the will to rally men and women to a common purpose and the character which inspires confidence.

—General Bernard Montgomery

In our national studies of quality improvement interventions, we found a sizable number of top leaders who devoted considerable time and energy to promoting quality improvement and patient safety initiatives. At one hospital, an infection preventionist reported that "several of our vice presidents . . . would actually go to the units and talk with the staff and see how [the initiative] was going." The reason was simple: In order to direct those in an organization on the right path, you have to first understand why they do the work the way they do it. As well, when a leader leaves the C-suite to meet with front-line staff and learn from them, it can inspire trust and respect for that leader's intentions and motivations.

On the other hand, we discovered hospitals that had completed very successful projects to reduce central line–associated bloodstream infection (CLABSI) and catheter-associated urinary tract infection (CAUTI) whose top executives did nothing more for the projects than refrain from rejecting them. The leadership came from elsewhere in the institution,

from physicians and nurses in every department and on every bureaucratic level. In these institutions, matters of safety were absorbed and led
by those on the front lines of care with little direction or intervention from
above. The power of an enthusiastic and well-respected nurse manager was
very often the secret sauce for a project's success when requiring changes
in nurse practice, and an engaging medical service chief filled a similar
role stimulating changes in physician practice. The importance of these
critical nurse or physician champions has too often been confirmed by
the negative impact their departures had on their respective interventions.

NONPROFITS ARE DIFFERENT

Surprisingly little has been written, in the popular media or in academe,
about leadership in a hospital setting. There has been a general assumption
that the best practices of leadership in business can be directly applied to
nonprofit institutions or that those in hospital leadership positions pos-
sess a vast amount of influence and power. Our research suggests otherwise, and we find that view supported by the business consultant and
author Jim Collins. In a monograph, *Good to Great and the Social Sectors*,
he contrasted the goals of the two worlds: "In the social sectors, the critical question is not, 'How much money do we make per dollar of invested
capital?' but, 'How effectively do we deliver on our mission and make a
distinctive impact, relative to our resources?'"[1]

That divergence has led to substantially different management
structures and roles. In for-profit corporations, the chief executive officer
(CEO) has the power to make decisions—on his own, if that's his style—
confident that his hierarchy will implement them. His leadership tends
to be transactional, ensuring that employee roles are clearly delineated
and motivating employees with punishments and rewards. But in such
institutions as universities, charities, and hospitals, the CEO and his or
her top aides must cope with a variety of independent power bases—
tenured professors, volunteers, physicians—who generally don't do well at
taking orders. The result, Collins said, is two distinct kinds of leadership

approaches. For-profit leaders, in general, exercise executive, command-and-control skills, whereas social sector leaders, if they want to succeed, must learn legislative skills such as the ability to communicate, listen, and persuade. Their leadership tends to be transformational rather than transactional, inspiring personnel to see beyond their immediate self-interest.[2] (See Box 6.1.)

The most successful hospital leaders, for example, are ambitious not so much for themselves or for the bottom line, Collins suggested, but for the institution's patient-centered mission. To effectively lead physicians, nurses, and other personnel who have a major personal stake in their life-saving profession, a leader, whatever her title, must share that motivation. The transformational leader adapts to the needs and motives of her followers and seeks to earn their trust. With their willing support, she can draw on the individual expertise and imagination so necessary to reaching and implementing the right decisions.

Box 6.1

TRANSACTIONAL VERSUS TRANSFORMATIONAL LEADERSHIP TRAITS[a]

Leadership Research: Transactional Versus Transformational

Transactional	Transformational
• Transaction (or exchange) of something the leader has that the follower wants	• Inspires followers to see beyond their self-interest
• Specifies roles and tasks	• Adapts to the needs and motives of followers
• Reward and punishment used as motivation	• Behaves in a way that engenders great trust
• "One size fits all"	• The leader often relies on charisma

[a]Adapted from Northouse.[2]

In his monograph, Collins described a meeting he had with a group of nonprofit healthcare leaders. As he had found in so many social sector sessions, the healthcare people obsessed about systemic constraints. "What needs to happen for you to build great hospitals?" he asked, and they responded with a litany of complaints about government, insurers, and patients. He advised them to move beyond simply focusing on their problems if they wanted to achieve greatness.

Fair enough, but the constraints on hospitals are, in fact, very considerable, and increasing. There's no question that they have a negative effect on leaders' attitudes and their behaviors toward proposed quality improvement initiatives.

Consolidation is roiling the profession. Mergers are creating ever more giant medical centers that threaten the existence of independent hospitals, while mergers among insurers have drained away much of hospitals' bargaining power. Hospitals' growing employment of physicians has substantially increased costs, often without matching increases in productivity. At the same time, the shortage of doctors is expected to reach 120,000 by 2030 according to the Association of American Medical Colleges.[3] The move toward electronic medical records continues to impose major financial burdens on hospitals and heavier workloads on healthcare workers. Government funding has dropped, as has Medicare reimbursement—and the list goes on.

In our research, we came upon hospital leaders who threw up their hands when "the system" put a roadblock in the way of progress. The chief quality officer at a major academically affiliated hospital told us that a quality improvement effort had been shot down by the clinical executive board with the comment, "Oh, no, we can't ask our residents to sign and date their orders within 24 hours." He blamed the decision on the department chair's inclination to favor academic priorities, such as writing papers and grants, and teaching, over clinical needs, and the quality officer dropped his proposal. At another site, the intensive care unit (ICU) director wanted to use a novel approach to reduce CLABSI in his unit because of an elevated infection rate and was stymied by the infection prevention staff. We asked why he didn't appeal the decision to someone in leadership. "You know," he said, "management changes so often . . . so that you kind of say, 'Well, is it worth working with them?' because if when you are done, you are just going to be starting all over again."

But effective leaders, we found, wherever they are in a hospital's hierarchy, don't take no for an answer. They find ways to accomplish their goals. The best C-suite leaders, for example, don't allow system challenges to keep them from their core mission—the cultivation of a culture of patient-centered clinical excellence.

There are innumerable definitions of leadership. Napoleon offered, "A leader is a dealer in hope." Lao Tzu, the ancient Chinese philosopher, said of the good leader, "When his work is done, his aim fulfilled, they will all say, 'We did this ourselves.'" We favor the straightforward definition of Peter G. Northouse, a preeminent scholar in leadership studies, from his book, *Leadership: Theory and Practice:* "Leadership is a process whereby an individual influences a group of individuals to achieve a common goal."[2] (See Box 6.2.)

Northouse described an invaluable distinction between two types of leadership. He called one "assigned leadership" because it is based on the position a person occupies in an organization. The other type he called

---

Box 6.2

KEY LEADERSHIP TRAITS[a]

Key Leadership Traits

- Persistence
- Intelligence
- Integrity
- Self-confidence
- Sociability

[a]Adapted from Northouse.[2]

"emergent leadership" because it emerges from an influential person in a group no matter what that person's position in the organization. In other words, you don't automatically become a leader because you're a manager. Warren Bennis and Burt Nanus put it succinctly in their book, *Leaders: Strategies for Taking Charge*: "Managers are people who do things right and leaders are people who do the right thing."[4]

THE ROLE OF HOSPITAL LEADERS

Hospital administrators and clinical chiefs can and should take on personal leadership roles in quality improvement initiatives. By simply mentioning a new infection prevention project as a reflection of the hospital's mission in their meetings and other encounters with staff members, they can help build powerful support for the project throughout the institution. They can stop by and listen to a reporting session on the initiative, boosting the team's sense of purpose. They can include updates on the project's progress in their hospital-wide newsletter and online communications. They can make the degree of a person's support of quality initiatives a regular element of employee performance reviews. And top supervisors can provide backing when those leading an initiative run up against immovable roadblocks. "We kind of have an open door to senior management if we need to," an infection preventionist told us, describing an initiative, "I mean, I can go up and talk to the chief of staff or the medical director or CEO of the hospital if I needed to."

The familiar and much-praised "management by walking around" leadership approach is effective if the leader is looking and listening and communicating his vision for the hospital. But too many leaders view management by walking around as an exercise in nitpicking, a chance to show how all-seeing and important they are. At one hospital, we encountered a chief of staff like that: He would spot a minor problem, insist that it be corrected instantly, and wait around for the correction, forcing staff members to ignore more pressing matters. In one case, the problem was a dirty corner, and he had everyone trying to reach the janitor to come clean it up.

Leaders do have to be hard-nosed, to hold their people accountable for results, but they need to pick their spots more carefully than that chief of staff. Though most problems yield to reason and compromise, some require a firm stand. Witness the familiar unwillingness of some physicians to fill out and complete medical records in a timely fashion. Many hospitals allow their physicians to bend the rules, afraid of antagonizing those who help to keep the beds full. Yet when hospitals get tough with, say, a leading surgeon to the point of suspending him for a week or two, the result is often beneficial: The surgeon returns ready to abide by the medical records policy, and his surgical colleagues (and other onlookers in different disciplines who may also be tardy) follow suit.

The chief of staff at an academically affiliated hospital gave us an example of her preference for dealing with problems head on, rather than letting them slide. One of her department heads received what she described as an "embarrassingly" poor audit score. She sat him down, read him the riot act, instructed him to improve his ways quickly—and sent a letter describing the situation to his university supervisor. The problem was soon resolved.

When there's staff turnover in a department, the boss faces mounting pressure to hire replacements rapidly because the remaining staff members are forced to take on extra duties. An infection preventionist leader we interviewed refused to fill a vacancy for a year because he wouldn't settle for second best. He was a strong advocate of the "hire hard, manage easy"[5] school of leadership. After finding the right person, he said, "My life is so much better." As the saying goes, "A's hire A's while B's hire C's."

PINPOINTING KEY LEADERSHIP BEHAVIORS

Some years ago, we studied 14 hospitals to see if we could identify the major characteristics of those leaders who were successful in implementing infection prevention practices.[6] We conducted 38 in-depth telephone interviews followed by 48 on-site interviews at six of the hospitals. The telephone interviews were with infection preventionists, hospital epidemiologists, infectious diseases physicians, and critical care nurse managers. The on-site interviews were primarily spread among the same group plus chief executives and directors, chairs and vice chairs of medicine, and quality managers or medical directors of quality. The following were the characteristics that stood out among those who led successful infection prevention projects, and they were confirmed in our more recent site visits and interviews (in total, we have studied 46 hospitals and conducted more than 450 interviews):

- They were dedicated to establishing or maintaining a culture of clinical excellence—and were successful at communicating that patient-centered vision to their staff. When physicians and nurses live by a culture that puts patient safety first, they are inevitably more open to infection prevention initiatives. At one of the hospitals we studied, when staff members came to the CEO with a disagreement, she would routinely ask, "What's the best thing for the patient?" That would settle the matter. And we saw indications that her philosophy had been absorbed by her staff.
- They were solution oriented, ready and able to overcome any and all barriers to success. Unlike those leaders quoted previously, who blamed the system for their inaction, effective leaders found answers. A hospital epidemiologist reported that his hospital had been getting nowhere with a CAUTI prevention project because of a lack of nursing leadership. Finally, he teamed up with nurse managers and nurses to conduct a successful initiative to reduce the use of Foleys. "We partnered with managers instead of nursing leaders," he said.
- They were inspirational, not only in articulating their vision, but also in leading other staff members to take on leadership roles. We encountered an outstanding example in the person of a hospital epidemiologist at a private hospital. "We're inspired having somebody like him," said the lead infection preventionist. "He's got that mindset. It's all about the safety of the patient . . . not getting caught up so much on the politics and

bureaucracy of it, just saying, 'OK, let's make this work.' That in itself energizes us."

- They were careful strategists, preparing the ground for a project, ready to do the preliminary politicking and to use their personal prestige to pave the way for acceptance. As a chief of medicine told us, "I think most hospitals . . . have too many committees and are less productive in terms of what they accomplish. If I'm going to take a serious vote at . . . a committee, I want to know the vote's results before they're taken." In another hospital, an infection preventionist, faced with an administrator who had turned down the purchase of large drapes for central line insertions, began by getting his proposal approved by the infection control committee and then built support among physicians. "They drive the bus," he said, "so that's why we partner with doctors all the time." When he went back to the administrator, he said, he was able to prove that he had examined other options, that he had the backing of the physicians who would use the equipment, and that the coverings were supported in the literature—and he got his drapes.

For leaders at any level within a hospital to bring about a successful quality improvement intervention, creating a new behavioral norm requires all those legislative skills that Jim Collins spoke of, and that includes a goodly helping of emotional intelligence.

Emotional intelligence—it became known as EQ, or emotional quotient, by analogy with IQ, for intelligence quotient—first came to public attention in an article by two psychologists, John Mayer and Peter Salovey, in 1997.[7] They defined it as the "ability to monitor one's own and others' feelings and emotions, to discriminate among them, and to use this information to guide one's thinking and action." The authors brought together a number of scientific discoveries of the time, some of them dealing with how the brain regulates emotions.

A leader's emotional intelligence is not just a matter of their being naturally friendly and sympathetic to other people, nor is it simply a knack for sensing what other people are feeling, though that's a part of it. EQ requires some degree of thinking about feelings, your own and those of others, and consciously using those emotions to help make decisions and solve problems. It calls for you to develop rules about emotions that can guide your behavior—anger often yields to shame, for example. And it encompasses the ability to manage emotions, your own and those of others, to achieve your goals. If you know that a colleague who has expressed his anger toward you is likely to be feeling somewhat ashamed of himself the next day, you know that he may welcome a chance to make up and reconsider his position. And you make sure they get that opportunity (tossing away your pride in order to salvage the relationship).

Thousands of schools around the world now teach EQ skills to students, and thousands of companies now apply emotional intelligence in judging whether to hire and promote employees and in training them to improve job performance. There is even a Consortium for Research on Emotional Intelligence in Organizations that aids companies, such as American Express and Johnson & Johnson, and government agencies, such as the Defense Finance Accounting Service, by improving their use of EQ. Studies have also shown that higher emotional intelligence among bedside nurses correlates with improved patient safety in regard to nosocomial complications such as infections and falls.[8]

THE FOLLOWERS' RESPONSIBILITY

A well-developed emotional intelligence can help leaders in so many ways, but all the various attributes of the successful hospital leader that we have discussed point to one essential goal: By definition, any leader must have followers. But until Robert E. Kelley came along with his *Harvard Business Review* article, "In Praise of Followers," in 1988,[9] nobody had bothered to give followers anything like the academic research accorded leaders— even though it's the followers who actually get the job done.

His first book[10] on the subject, *The Power of Followership*, in 1992, was a bestseller. When he began his work on followership, he wrote, "I felt like the odd person out. Executives, academics, and even people sitting next to me on airplanes questioned why I would bother with followership when leadership spurred the media attention, research funding, and high-paying corporate gigs. . . . At some point, I finally decided to put a stake in the ground."

Kelley identified five key types of followers:

- Alienated. They are mavericks who may be capable, but they tend to be highly cynical, and they have a healthy skepticism toward the organization.
- Conformists. They are the organization's "yes people," but they generally exercise limited independent thinking.
- Passivists. They lack initiative and any sense of responsibility. They require disproportionate supervision relative to their contribution.
- Pragmatists. They hug the middle of the road. They will do a good job but won't stick their necks out.
- Exemplary followers. They manage themselves and their work well, constantly improving their skills. They have a commitment to the organization and its vision. They are innovative and independent, willing to question their leaders.

As you may have noted, that description of exemplary followers bears a strong resemblance to our earlier description of successful leaders. As Kelley wrote, "Instead of seeing the leadership role as superior to and more active than the role of the follower, we can think of them as equal but different activities." Other researchers went on to claim that followership was itself a form of leadership, a skill set that could be and should be taught as a leadership requirement.[10]

Leaders intent on reducing infection may be interested to learn that a recent survey[11] of infection preventionists indicated that the vast majority (73%) of followers are categorized as "exemplary" based on a combination of high scores in the domains of active engagement and independent thinking. Exemplary followership was associated with increased odds of regularly using urinary catheter reminders or stop orders or nurse-initiated urinary catheter discontinuation. Hospitals with the most exemplary followers were more likely to routinely use critical infection prevention strategies.

Leaders should sit down with each of their immediate followers and explain the mission and vision of the organization. They need to describe what the follower's role is and how that role contributes to the mission. By the time the meeting is over, the follower should understand the standards by which his or her performance will be measured. And for their followers to achieve their full potential, leaders should schedule regular individual catch-up sessions every month or so. That's how followers can be helped to become exemplary followers.

In the hospital setting, of course, some of the attributes of good followership are already in place. Most staff members in any hospital share a commitment to the institution and to the hospital's patient-centered vision. (Consider the clinical pharmacist who was monitoring adherence to the sedation and weaning protocols during an initiative to prevent ventilator-associated pneumonia at a hospital we studied. Unasked, he added head-of-bed elevation to the list of items he was checking. That's good followership.) As for being independent and willing to question leaders, that comes naturally to physicians and to at least some nurses.

THE POWER OF THE GROUP

When a hospital's leaders initiate a quality improvement intervention, however, they confront a daunting challenge. They must convince enough followers to alter their habitual way of proceeding in order to tip the balance of the institution toward a new set of habits. One of the greatest stumbling blocks in that process is the emotional weight of old habits—the old norm. Just because a leader asks them, followers don't willingly give up their norm. They are more likely to change their ways, though, if a new process gains a certain level of group approval.

That phenomenon is bred in our bones. Animal research has demonstrated the power of group norms. In a study of wild vervet monkeys,[12] for example, four groups were each presented with adjacent trays, blue-dyed corn in one, pink-dyed corn in the other. The colors were carefully chosen to attract the attention of both sexes—they represent the colors of the vervet's testicles. In two of the groups, the blue was more bitter-tasting than the pink and vice versa for the other two groups. The members of all four groups opted for the more tasteful corn, regardless of its color, creating group preferences. Four months later, after a new cohort of infants matured enough for solid foods, the trays were put back in place, but this time neither the blue nor the pink corn was bitter-tasting. The infants overwhelmingly partook of the corn color their mothers ate. But when 10 adult male members of the four groups migrated to settle in new groups, they found that their new group favored corn of a different color from their original choice—and they switched to the local color, even though their association with that color had been negative. The power of the group norm outweighed their personal norm.

Yet it is specifically a group norm—the traditional attitudes and procedures for dealing with Foleys, central venous catheters, and mechanical ventilators—that the quality initiatives discussed in this book must overcome. The outstanding scholar of how that can happen, of how innovation spreads, is Everett M. Rogers, who was born on his family's farm in Iowa in 1931 and grew up expecting to follow in his father's footsteps. A visit to Iowa State University changed his mind, and he eventually earned a PhD there in sociology and statistics.

In 1962, Rogers published *Diffusion of Innovations*. It describes the process whereby a new idea is accepted by a group or social system, starting with the innovators, who represent just 2.5% of the group. The idea begins to get a foothold with the early adopters (13.5%). It speeds up as it captures the early majority (about a third), and triumphs with the late majority (again, about a third). All that's left, then, is to wrap up the laggards (16%).[13]

Sometimes, the laggards take some convincing. When Rogers was a child, his father decided not to plant the then-new hybrid seed corn, which was said to be drought resistant and had been adopted by a neighboring farmer. When a devastating drought struck Iowa that year, the Rogers's corn wilted while the neighbor's crop flourished. The next year, Rogers senior planted the hybrid.

The diffusion of an idea or innovation, Rogers said, "is essentially a process occurring through interpersonal networks." He tracked an individual's reactions to an idea or innovation through various stages, from her first exposure to the idea, to her active interest in learning more about it, to her deciding to try it to determine how useful or desirable it is, to her final adoption. All sorts of influences can affect that process, from political rallies to TV ads, but the reactions and experiences of the members of the individual's group are key.

When we have to make a decision, we listen to the advice of our families and friends and neighbors—the people we trust. If they buy a particular brand of refrigerator or car, if they are signing on to a new medical plan, we're inclined to follow suit. It just makes sense that people who are like us will be good guides. Their reactions to ideas and innovations are going to be similar to what ours would be since, after all, that's part of what makes us all members of the same group, the same social system. And in any event, it's just more comfortable to be doing what the majority of our group's members do.

No, we're not in the same class as the vervet monkeys, certainly not in the same genetics class—but the general principle holds just as true for us. Though leaders can lean us in one or another direction, we tend to go along with the group consensus when confronted by an innovation. We trust the group.

In most cases, the arrival of an innovation, like a quality improvement initiative, forces us to contemplate changing the way we live in some way, large or small. Often, our reaction is annoyance. We don't want to be bothered; we're doing very nicely without the new device or idea.

So, Rogers asked, if you want to convince a group of people, many of them resistant, to accept a new idea or initiative, what's the most productive approach? His answer is this: Find members of the group who are generally admired and trusted and who believe in the new idea or initiative—and set them loose on the group as a whole. They are by far the best leaders for any kind of change. "Example is not the main thing in influencing others," Albert Schweitzer said, "it is the only thing."

And that is why most infection prevention initiatives today, like those we describe at the model hospital, rely so heavily on person-to-person contacts between members of a project team and the hospital staff. A physician champion is the natural person to convince other physicians to alter their attitudes toward the Foley, for example. A nurse champion is the natural person to convince other nurses that Foleys cause infection and should be removed with alacrity. Yes, the champions must be chosen with care. If the physician champion selected is unpopular with his colleagues or unknown to most of them, he is unlikely to get the job done. If the nurse champion lacks a warm and friendly personality, she is unlikely to inspire her colleagues to change their ways. But these caveats aside, the evidence of hundreds of initiatives supports the Rogers premise as the most efficient approach to revising a hospital's clinical norms.

That said, the hospital leadership still has an important responsibility in any initiative. As suggested previously, the administrative and clinical leaders need to be supportive of the project, using their bully pulpit within the organization. Our studies do suggest that, although the administrative side may be very helpful, the major leadership burden often falls on the clinical leaders, both nursing and physician leadership. If they are not engaged in visibly supporting an initiative, if they are not responsive to appeals from project leaders, if they are not respected within the hospital community, quality initiatives often flounder.

We have also found that hospitals whose leaders, administrative as well as clinical, have created or maintained a culture of excellence are likely to have successful quality initiatives. That's because such hospitals allow project champions to grow and flourish and because the sites accept such initiatives as opportunities for improvement.

At the hospital mentioned previously, where the pharmacist took on an extra monitoring task, we learned how a variety of leaders can bring a quality improvement initiative to fruition. The initial impetus for the project came from the chief operating officer, who announced that the hospital was going to adopt standards from the highly regarded Institute for Healthcare Improvement (a nonprofit organization founded by Donald Berwick that has championed patient safety initiatives throughout the world). That inspired nursing leadership to consider ventilator-associated pneumonia prevention. The Critical Care Nurse Practice Committee picked up the leadership ball, reviewing the literature, and deciding that the chief point of attack would be bed elevation—making sure that the head of the bed of patients on a ventilator was at an elevation of at least 30 degrees to reduce the chance of aspiration.

A critical care nurse manager was a leader on the floor, organizing in-services, putting up educational posters, and talking up the initiative with colleagues. At the same time, this nurse champion monitored beds herself for six months. The hospital's overworked infection control staff was supportive but not actively involved in the project, though they were enthusiastic observers—"jumping up and down" about it, a nurse reported. Top-level management was not involved either. The project leaders were a nurse manager and a handful of other nurses, and when the initiative led to a drastic reduction in the incidence of pneumonia among patients on ventilators, it was the nurse managers and the bedside nurses on the floor who deserved the credit.

In the next chapter, we look at the problems encountered during the implementation of a quality improvement intervention, including a rogues' gallery of the three kinds of staff members who are responsible for most of those problems: active resisters, organizational constipators, and time-servers. We offer suggestions for coping with each of them.

SUGGESTIONS FOR FURTHER READING

Blackshear PB. The followership continuum: a model for increasing organizational productivity. The Innovation Journal: The Public Sector Innovation Journal. 2004;9:article 7.

   In this article, the author presented the stages of followership within a model for measuring workforce performance level that he referred to as the Followership Continuum. The author proposed that, by focusing on assessing and developing the highest followership stages of the continuum, workforce productivity can be greatly improved.

Blanchard K, Johnson S. The One Minute Manager. 3rd ed. New York, NY: Morrow; 2003.
   One of the most widely read management books, *The One Minute Manager* tells the story of a young man on a quest to "find out what really [makes] an effective manager tick." Through this concise, easy-to-read story, advice is shared in the form of three extremely practical "secrets": one minute goals; one minute praisings; and one minute reprimands.

Brown B. Dare to Lead. New York, NY: Random House; 2018.
   This book shares recent research learned from the leaders of organizations small and large about their courageous journeys as change-makers and culture shifters.

Greene MT, Saint S. Followership characteristics among infection preventionists in US hospitals: results of a national survey. Am J Infect Control. 2016;44:343–345.
   In this 2013 survey completed by 403 infection preventionists in the United States, 73% of lead infection preventionists were classified as exemplary followers. Regular use of key prevention practices was variable, but hospitals with the most exemplary followers were more likely to routinely employ several recommended practices, such as urinary catheter reminders and stop orders.

Kelley R. In Praise of Followers: Harvard Business Review; 1988. Accessed November 24, 2020 at https://hbr.org/1988/11/in-praise-of-followers
   In this article, the author argued that organizations stand or fall because of not only how well their leaders lead, but also how well their followers follow. Although many management books explore the traits necessary to be a strong leader, Kelley explored those necessary to encourage effective following.

Northouse PG. Leadership: Theory and Practice. 8th ed. Thousand Oaks, CA: Sage; 2018.
   Used as the standard textbook at colleges and universities worldwide, this book is an accessible presentation of the major theories and models of leadership. The author included practical exercises and case studies throughout. A must-have for anyone interested in the topic.

Saint S, Chopra V. Thirty Rules for Healthcare Leaders. Ann Arbor, MI: Michigan Publishing Services; 2019.
   This book provides brief pearls of wisdom specifically geared toward those in healthcare. Intended for all roles in healthcare—regardless of title or experience— and designed for the time-pressured individual, each rule provides practical advice that can be put to use immediately.

Saint S, Kowalski CP, Banaszak-Holl J, Forman J, Damschroder L, Krein SL. The importance of leadership in preventing healthcare-associated infection: results of a multisite qualitative study. Infect Control Hosp Epidemiol. 2010;31:901–907.
   In this article, Saint and colleagues followed up on preliminary data that indicated that hospital leadership played an important role in whether a hospital was engaged in infection prevention activities. They found that successful leaders (1) cultivated a culture of clinical excellence and effectively communicated it to staff; (2) focused on overcoming barriers and dealt directly with resistant staff or process issues that impeded prevention of healthcare-associated infection; (3) inspired their employees; and (4) thought strategically while acting locally, which involved politicking before

crucial committee votes, leveraging personal prestige to move initiatives forward, and forming partnerships across disciplines.

Sinek S. Start With Why: How Great Leaders Inspire Everyone to Take Action. New York, NY: Portfolio by Penguin Group; 2011.

This book describes the idea of the Golden Circle to explain why some leaders are more influential, inspiring, and innovative than others to generate loyalty, team success, and even social movements.

Common Problems, Realistic Solutions

First they ignore you. Then they laugh at you. Then they fight you. And then... you win.

—Mohandas k. Gandhi

The nurse manager was an enthusiastic supporter of the bladder bundle, but her plans were opposed by the hospital's nurse executive. "She's a very energetic person and loves to try new things," the nurse executive said. "She doesn't realize it's not her kitchen so she can't make a new cake every day." In this case, the ill-fated "cake" happened to be a prevention initiative focused on catheter-associated urinary tract infection (CAUTI).

There are two basic kinds of problems to be resolved in undertaking a project to prevent healthcare-associated infections (HAIs). Some barriers are of a practical, technical nature, the natural consequence of disrupting a system as complex as a hospital—new physicians' orders must be developed, bedside carts must be reconfigured. Other barriers are more personal in nature: the resistance of physicians, nurses, and administrators to a change they don't like because it's seen as mistaken or inconvenient or, as in the case of that nurse executive, because it is seen as challenging authority and the status quo. In this chapter, we explore both kinds of problems and offer some best practice ideas for coping with them.

When we last visited our model, 250-bed hospital, the bladder bundle initiative on 4 West had been a success. Now, the administration has decided to go global, to carry the initiative to the institution as a whole. The elements of the bundle and the implementation approach will remain the same, including the daily catheter patrol, for example. But the major expansion of the intervention is generating substantial new challenges.

One of the reasons 4 West was chosen to pilot the intervention was the positive attitude its leaders and bedside nurses had exhibited toward earlier improvement efforts. Now, the project leaders will have to cope with the full gamut of staff reactions, the total range of emotional responses in more than a dozen different units and departments. At the same time, the demands on various parts of the hospital will increase. For example, the supply department will start receiving multiple requests for condom catheters or bladder scanners, and the infection prevention department will have to organize and analyze copious new reams of data.

The intervention will also require a somewhat new leadership structure, though no such change might be needed in a smaller facility. Our executive sponsor will stay on, as will the project manager—a major advantage since the lessons the manager learned and the contacts she made dealing with 4 West will be a substantial help in coordinating the hospital-wide rollout. The nurse and physician champions are taking on new roles in the intervention as the go-to people for their counterparts throughout the hospital; there will be a nurse champion for each unit on the medical floor as well as a nurse and physician champion for the emergency department and each intensive care unit (ICU). In that way, the project leaders hope to be able to tailor the intervention to the particularities of the various units. One unit, for example, might have an unusually large percentage of patients who are incontinent, leading the team to arrange for extra nursing assistance.

Any quality improvement enterprise can encounter a variety of baked-in challenges. The big teaching hospitals are slow moving and bureaucratic, with a tendency to consider themselves special, as in, "our floor patients are so sick they'd be in the ICU at any other hospital." Their tenured faculty members are often less interested in clinical matters, such as quality initiatives, than they are in research, the primary track for promotion. A few examples of the barriers that exist include the following:

- Cutbacks in personnel and physical resources may have already strained clinical staff, so an emergency department might rule out the use of intermittent straight catheters as Foley alternatives because of the extra nursing time required.
- Existing organizational policies can conflict with the recommendations of the intervention. An obstetrics department order, for instance, may call for the automatic placement of an indwelling catheter for every patient receiving epidural analgesia.
- Rigid employment rules make it difficult to remove uncooperative or underperforming personnel. As one infection preventionist sarcastically put it, "You don't get fired if you work for this outfit; well, maybe if you kill four people and they find three of the bodies."
- Each project has to compete with other quality initiatives for staff time and resources, and these initiatives are proliferating.
- Some physicians are going to resist any kind of new technology, including the electronic patient records system.
- Passive resistance can be a challenge, as when team members agree to changes during meetings, providing all the desired responses, but then fail to follow through on making the changes.

In what follows, we have provided a list of common barriers and possible solutions that hospitals have found successful. (See Table 7.1.)

Staff misunderstandings can be a major obstacle to a successful quality improvement intervention. For instance, the bladder bundle accepts the use of an indwelling catheter for prolonged immobilization, say for a patient with a lumbar spine fracture. We encountered nurses who interpreted that to mean that they should use a Foley for patients on bed rest. Some hospitals found that using the condom catheter instead of the Foley was problematic since the condom catheter chosen rarely stayed on the male patient. The constant leakage of urine on the patient's bedsheets

Table 7.1 Barriers and Solutions

Barriers to Successful Intervention	Possible Solutions
Some nurses may not be on board with indwelling urinary catheter removal	• Get buy-in before implementation. For example, ask, "Whom do we have to convince on this floor?" Have that person help to develop the plan or participate in the education for that unit.
	• Listen to nurses' concerns and address them to nurses' satisfaction.

Lack of or problems with nurse champions	• Identify the types of champions who work in your organization. Do not use a one-size-fits-all strategy. For example,
	  • Use nurse educators or charge nurses or unit managers as champions.
	  • Have more than one nurse champion (i.e., co-champions).

	• Recognize nurse champions via such mechanisms as certificates of recognition, annual evaluation appraisals, newsletters, and notifying the nursing director.
Lack of physician buy-in of new practices	• Provide data to physicians about urinary catheter use, monthly indwelling urinary catheter prevalence, and CAUTI rates.
	• Provide one-on-one education (evidence based and safety oriented).
	• Engage medical leadership support—by the chief of staff, for example.
	• Involve physicians as much as possible in planning, education, and implementation; include physicians on your team.
	• Identify a physician champion who will • Meet with other physicians to get them on board.

Table 7.1 CONTINUED

Barriers to Successful Intervention	Possible Solutions
	• Back up nurses when there's a disagreement.
	• Present evidence such as highlighting how often physicians who have patients with indwelling urinary catheters forget about them.
Lack of physician champion	• In institutions where there are good nurse–physician working relationships, most physicians may be willing to go along with recommendations by nurses, especially if the new practice is viewed as a "nursing initiative."
	• Also see previous discussion about overcoming resistant physicians.
Leadership does not see CAUTI as a priority	• Prepare and present a business case to help convince leadership that the time and cost factors for implementing the new practice will be worth it.
	• Be sure leadership receives monthly CAUTI rates and catheter use data.
General guidance	• Get people on the team who feel CAUTI is worth addressing.
	• Highlight staff who have adopted the new practice.
	• Know the system and how to get practice changes through relevant committees.
Inflexible nurse schedules make education in new practices difficult	• Rather than having the nurses attend education sessions, bring the education to the bedside. Do competencies on the unit, talking with nurses one to one during the point prevalence assessments.
	• Incorporate education on CAUTI into annual competency testing.

(*continued*)

Table 7.1 CONTINUED

Barriers to Successful Intervention	Possible Solutions
Nurses are not confident speaking with physicians about removal	• Find a physician champion to support nurse requests for removal.
	• Have the nurse manager prompt nurses to speak with physicians.
	• Provide education on communication.
Surgeon and urologist resistance to early removal of indwelling urinary catheter	• Have the physician champion present at a medical staff meeting about indications and nonindications for indwelling urinary catheters.
	• Work with the physician assistants to discontinue indwelling urinary catheters within 1 or 2 days after surgery.
	• Engage a surgeon and/or urologist as a physician champion and work with that person to establish conditions under which the catheter can be removed.

and gown—caused by a substandard product or improper placement technique—led to unhappy patients and unhappy nurses.

Efforts to reduce infection rates can also be sabotaged by the inadequate training or proficiency of those who are placing the Foleys and straight catheters. One nurse executive had occasion to evaluate competencies of a group of nurses' aides: "I had a mannequin down there, and what I saw was kind of scary." Nurses' aides trained by registered nurses (RNs) would, in turn, train new aides, and errors would compound. In that hospital, aides and RNs now refresh their catheter insertion skills annually, using real people as well as mannequins.

In addition to monitoring the reactions of the staff to a quality initiative, the project leaders need to keep a wary eye on their own team. A nurse champion with a patronizing attitude toward bedside nurses can under-mine the most carefully planned project. And beware of the team member who always explains away unexpected personnel problems as the result of staff resistance, a scapegoating technique to divert attention from his or her own mistakes. It's important for the team as a whole to remember that resistance, for all its annoyance, can sometimes be extremely valu-able, signaling a weakness in the project that requires correction—or a special circumstance that demands an exception to the recommendations of the bladder bundle.

Leaders of change efforts of any kind need to keep in mind the power of positive deviance, an approach to problem-solving that looks for those outliers in every community whose tendency to avoid status quo thinking and behavior can reveal important new solutions for the community as a whole.[1] The positive deviance approach was first applied in the 1990s in Vietnam villages where the majority of children suffered from malnu-trition. A handful of outlier families with well-nourished children was studied. They were found to be feeding their children foods that the other families viewed as inappropriate for children, including shrimp and sweet potato greens. Once the community was convinced to try that diet, the malnutrition faded.

One hospital with an eye for outliers may create a special committee when it is about to scale up an intervention. The committee would consist of physicians and nurses with a reputation for criticizing such projects. At meetings, the committee members are urged to report what they see as problems in the proposed intervention, and the project leaders take careful notes. Along with the expected knee-jerk complaints, the leaders generally uncover some real shortcomings. As an added benefit, the fault-finding members of the committee, having vented their views, tend to maintain a neutral position toward the intervention once it is underway.[2]

The most important single factor in any such project, of course, is the quality of the individual hospital's culture. It's a word that has been greatly devalued, its meaning stretched beyond recognition, but to paraphrase Justice Potter Stewart's famous comment about pornography, we know a dysfunctional culture when we see it. The staff members are territorial rather than supportive; averse to change rather than invested in their unit's efficiency; obedient rather than empowered; extrinsically, rather than intrinsically, motivated. Quality interventions are unlikely to flourish in such arid soil.

In the day-to-day operation of a quality improvement project, the leaders' greatest challenge is to convince the clinical staff to adopt new goals and practices. In our view, there are three types of staff members who present the most problems for an initiative: (1) active resisters openly oppose the intervention; (2) organizational "constipators" get in the way; and (3) time-servers undermine it by reason of their very laziness and indifference. We discuss them next in that same sequence, in emotionally descending order. The time-servers are the most difficult to convert into project supporters.

ACTIVE RESISTERS

Physicians and nurses among the active resisters often cite similar reasons for their attitude, including a shared distaste for any project that rocks the boat, as in, "If it ain't broke, don't fix it." However, the underlying reasons for their opposition, the ways in which it manifests, and the best responses to their behavior are often different, enough so that we believe the two groups warrant separate treatment.[3]

The most extreme emergence of the resistant physician takes place during an encounter between a physician and a nurse during rounds outside a patient's room, by a patient's bed, or on a telephone. The nurse says something like, "Dr. Jones, according to the bladder bundle, I think the Foley should be removed," and Dr. Jones replies, "After you go to medical school, Miss Smith, you can tell me what to do." More than one staff member has told us that story, and others have the physician saying, "You are just a nurse. Don't question me," or, "Who asked you?"

That sounds as though the physicians' motivations had more to do with their ego than anything else—as they viewed it, their judgment and practice had been challenged—and certainly ego plays a role. Physicians have traditionally been trained to see themselves as independent and self-regulating, the ultimate authority charged with life-saving responsibility. They do not expect to be monitored or corrected in their medical practice, certainly not by a nonphysician in front of other hospital personnel.

Yet there can be a variety of other reasons behind their resistance to a quality initiative. In some cases, a different kind of embarrassment may be at play because the physicians simply did not know that their patient even had a Foley or had forgotten it was there. One study[4] found that attending physicians were unaware that their patient had an indwelling catheter 38% of the time, and the inappropriate catheters were more often missed than the appropriate ones. Many inappropriate Foleys remain in place until there is some complication related to the catheters or until just before the patients are discharged. It's not just true for Foleys. Studies of vascular catheters—peripherally inserted central catheters (PICCs) and central lines—have similarly found that one in five physicians were unaware that their patient had this type of device.[5]

Physicians in general, and surgeons in particular, sometimes oppose an intervention because of a tendency to be paranoid by profession. Any kind of change, they fear, will throw them off their game and threaten the modus operandi they have so carefully developed, with possibly dire consequences for both patient and physician. Resident physicians don't want to risk straying beyond what they've just been taught.

As suggested previously, physicians may also resist quality improvement interventions because they are doubters: They have seen too many new theories disproven, too many "revolutionary" new techniques abandoned. Reports of fraud in scientific studies have become all too familiar. And they simply don't believe that all of the changes required by the intervention are scientifically valid or necessary. Indeed, as discussed in Chapter 3, some of the items in the bladder bundle are based more on common sense and observational studies than on rigorous randomized controlled trials. Physicians also have a tendency to view a quality initiative as research rather than as real medical practice. They see a research project as temporary, to be ignored until it disappears, while they get on with the serious work.

Underlying the opposition of some physicians—and nurses, as well—
is their conviction that catheters and urinary tract infections represent
an inferior order of medical problem. Why, they wonder, are we being
pestered about such a minor matter when we are battling cancer, heart disease, and the like? A qualitative study found that a number of physicians
interviewed simply did not believe that CAUTI posed a significant risk to
their patients, particularly when compared to such infections as central
line-associated bloodstream infection (CLABSI). As a result, CAUTI prevention was not a priority.[6]

At one institution, as the CAUTI intervention was starting, the hospital
leadership decided that a urinary catheter reminder linked to a physician's
order for a urinary catheter should be developed to engage doctors in the
project. The staff member assigned that task first went to check out the
institution's catheter policy in general—and discovered that there was
none. Physicians who wanted Foleys placed gave verbal instructions to
the nurses and didn't even bother to write orders for the catheters.

Resistance by older physicians was especially problematic at one small,
rural hospital. A director of quality described her institution as "the Rip
Van Winkle of hospitals." The physicians, she said, have a "captain of the
ship mentality." And when the "cash cow" surgeon refused to abide by the
bladder bundle, she added, "Do you think anybody is going to hold him
accountable?"

In fact, hospitals have traditionally looked on doctors as their
customers—they who bring in the patients—but that has been changing.
Many leading hospitals today are reshaping that relationship. They see patient care as more team based than doctor centered, with the nurse a full
partner. They are demanding that physicians join them in treating the patient as the new customer in chief and support the innovations that serve
that customer's safety. Younger independent physicians and hospitalists
are more likely to have heard and accepted that message than older
practitioners.

At our model hospital, physicians who ignore bladder bundle practices
because they doubt their scientific validity find themselves collared by
the project's physician champion in the physicians' lounge or after a staff

meeting. They are shown scientific studies describing the impressive drop in infections following bladder bundle interventions, especially after the timely removal of Foleys. They are shown statistics on the substantial incidence of CAUTI in their own hospital, including its financial impact. Finally, the physician champion acknowledges that there is always some element of risk in adopting a new policy, but he challenges the resister physician by asking, in effect, "How about the risk to your patients if you don't go along with the change?"

Each weekday of the first weeks of the hospital-wide intervention at the model hospital, the bedside nurses on catheter patrol indicate on the template and on the paper chart the status of their patients' Foleys, including why they are in place. If an appropriate indication is not identified, they inform the physician that it is time to remove the Foley. Whether that is done in person or on a telephone, the intervention calls for that contact to be made each day an inappropriate Foley is present. And even for a habitual physician resister, that can have an effect. A bedside nurse told us, "The doctors catch on after a while. They get sick of listening to us, and they don't like phone calls."

Early in the intervention at the model hospital, as a way of easing doctors and nurses into the changes, a catheter reminder has been attached to the physician notes on patients' charts, on paper and in the electronic record. As noted previously, this low-cost system calls the physician's attention to the Foley and includes the basic components of the bladder bundle. Reminders can be effective, but one warning: It's so easy to add them to the computer system that there is danger of reminder overload. Hospitals need to develop ways to prioritize reminders in order to keep them under control.

After a week of reminders, when there is still some physician resistance, the model hospital posts a 48-hour default stop order for each Foley, indicating when it should be removed. The name of the hospital's medical director is prominently displayed on the order to further encourage cooperation. The stop order appears on patients' paper charts and on computerized patient records, and, when the date arrives, the template generates an electronic alert. In addition to the two kinds of reminders, some hospitals, faced with uncooperative doctors, have required physicians to sign plastic tape flags attached to the reminder sheets, indicating that they have been made aware of the bladder bundle requirements. Those who failed to do so were sent alphanumeric pages—a much more intrusive step, and a forceful reminder of a reminder.

In many hospitals, if not most, a doctor's order is required before a nurse is allowed to remove a Foley. As a result, when a nurse observes that a Foley should come out according to the bladder bundle standard, she must reach out to the physician until she finds him, even if it takes hours or days. We believe that is too long a time and too dangerous a policy. If there is any substantial delay, the nurse should be empowered to remove the catheter.

In its negotiations with resisting physicians, the project team at the model hospital treats them with respect and consideration and an appeal to their collegiality. Team members constantly remind each other that the majority of doctors and nurses, including the active resisters, have gone into healthcare to help people, certainly not to harm them. One project manager likes to recall an experiment in which three different signs were placed at a hospital's handwashing stations over a two-week period.[7] One sign said that washing would keep the user from catching diseases, the second said washing would keep patients from catching diseases, and a third sign, serving as a control, had a generic message. Compared with the other signs, the patient-oriented sign inspired a 33% increase in the quantity of disinfectant and soap used at each station.

Eventually, with a handful of doctors still resisting the intervention, and expressing their opposition openly on rounds and at staff meetings, the model hospital's project team decides it needs topside help. The physician champion and project manager appeal to the hospital's medical director, and he agrees to send a stiff email to each of the holdouts demanding their cooperation. If that fails, the hospital's administrative and clinical leaders have decided they will give the offenders a stark choice: Cease their resistance or leave the hospital. If the patient is, in fact, the customer, they agree, the hospital cannot continue to tolerate physicians who will not put the patient's safety first.

Nurses become active resisters because they, like their physician counterparts, prefer the status quo, but their motivations are very different. Many of the resisters are veteran nurses who have spent their careers using the Foley both to lighten their workload and as a convenient tool for measuring urinary flow. They have, for example, used Foleys in patients who urinate frequently. As one nurse put it, "Some of the ladies go maybe 100 cc every 15 to 20 minutes, and you're in there constantly answering the lights." The resisters insist that the Foley alternatives, such as frequently toileting the ambulatory patients or using bedpans, take precious time away from other patients who may have greater need of their care. The impact of these longtime nurse resisters is compounded because they are the people to whom new and younger nurses go for advice.

For some nurse resisters, their main complaint centers on the need to alert physicians about the requirements of the bladder bundle for patients with Foleys. Some of these nurses insist that the decision to use or not use a Foley is the business of the physician, not the nurse's responsibility. Others find it impossible to challenge physicians under any circumstances.

There are other aspects of the intervention that stir nurses' opposition because they increase the workload. Collecting data on Foley use, for example, can be complicated and time consuming. In hospitals without an electronic database, paper records must be gone through. Sometimes catheterizations go undocumented, so the catheter patrol has to check under each patient's bed sheets. Determining whether a patient has a urinary tract infection can also be a lengthy process. A positive urine culture, for example, may or may not be definitive depending on whether the patient meets a set of qualifying symptoms—symptoms that can vary depending on the patient's age and ailments. If the patient is immunocompromised, for instance, she may not spike a fever with an infection.

Supporting the nurses' opposition is their general belief that urinary tract infection is not a serious concern. "Let's think about it," an infection preventionist said. "The majority of our RNs are still female, and they've had hundreds of urinary tract infections in their lifetime. They did not die." In fact, they simply took narrow-spectrum antimicrobials, and the problem went away. We found that attitude to be all but universal in the hospitals we studied. When a patient falls, a clinical executive told us, he dispatches aides to get all the facts, to check procedures on every shift, to call meetings. "But if we get a Foley infection," he continued, "nobody says, 'Oooo, let's have a huddle and see how it happened.'"

The nurses' opposition to the project takes several forms. Sometimes they simply ignore the initiative, asking physicians to order a Foley regardless of whether it meets the bladder bundle appropriateness criteria or failing to speak to physicians about its timely removal. They may neglect to share information about patients with Foleys with their counterparts at shift change. They may also find ways to game the system.

The electronic medical records, for all their efficiency, provide opportunities for a workaround. Some hospitals use a scoring algorithm to help determine whether a catheter should be removed. Nurse resisters know what number is needed to make it appear that the catheter should stay in place, and use it rather than the number appropriate to the particular patient. In other hospitals, the electronic checklist of approved indications for ordering a catheter (or for keeping one in place) is followed by an "other" category. Resister nurses and doctors connive in checking that category when, in fact, there is no medical reason to place a Foley or to keep one in place.

We learned of one hospital that seemed to be doing well with a bladder bundle intervention on most counts, but then officials noticed that there was a strange surge in the number of cases of bladder outlet obstruction, at least as reflected in the reasons cited for maintaining a Foley on the medical records template. The officials concluded that the intervention might not be going as well as they thought.

At the model hospital, the project team has developed some specific solutions for individual problems posed by nurse resisters. It has eliminated the nurse–physician confrontation over removal of a Foley by empowering nurses to take out the catheter as called for by the bladder bundle without obtaining the physician's approval. In units with a larger-than-usual ratio of patients who urinate frequently, "small zones" have been established so that nurses who had been responsible for nine such patients were now responsible for seven. In other units where nurses have been feeling harried because of the intervention, nurses' aides are now instructed to devote more of their time to toileting patients. Hourly rounding has been instituted, which saves nurses time in the long run. (In our experience, when nurses say a patient needs to urinate every 15 minutes, it's generally an exaggeration—it just seems that short a time!)

The model hospital has also sought ways to make the right thing to do the easy thing to do, integrating each new quality improvement project with earlier safety initiatives. The hourly rounds for the bladder bundle intervention, for instance, were compatible with an intervention aimed at preventing falls. We learned of another hospital where a project on pressure ulcers accommodated the bladder bundle: The use of absorbent pads and external urinary catheters for men and women as part of their skin protection and pressure ulcer initiative served as helpful alternatives for catheter use for incontinence concerns.

To create a more positive culture around the intervention, a team effort, the hospital has posted the Foley prevalence rate and CAUTI rates on boards in all the units, showing nurses the results of their work. Those who are cooperating with the project are recognized with praise and assured that their good work will be included in annual staff evaluations. Staff meeting time is set aside to report on the progress and challenges of the initiative.

Nurse champions spend one-on-one time with resisters, often putting less emphasis on bringing down the hospital's CAUTI rates and more on the benefits of the bladder bundle for the nurses' patients—the discomfort and possible internal injury of the Foley versus the chance to get up and around and out of the hospital sooner. The appeal is to the nurse resister's dedication to her patients' welfare.

Before moving on to discuss organizational constipators and time-servers, we should mention another species of active resister: the patient and/or the patient's family. Patients who are worried about soiling themselves or who want to stay in bed will appeal to their physicians and nurses to maintain a Foley in place, even when it is not needed. And the device is so routine and of secondary concern for the clinical staff that they will often go along. "You know what," a physician told an infection preventionist, "they're laying there. They're miserable and they want the Foley. So, let them have it." Families also sometimes request a Foley because they worry the patient will fall if he or she leaves the bed. This adage also holds true (perhaps more so) for vascular catheters. Patients often say, "I have terrible veins and had a PICC placed last time; why can't I get one this time around?" After all, no one likes to be treated like a pincushion, and patients who have experienced the comfort associated with having a ready source for blood draws often don't want to go back.

At the model hospital, nurses are trained to explain to patients about the potential discomfort and damage urinary and vascular catheters can cause, including a false feeling of the need to urinate and blood clots or infection. They emphasize the efficiency of Foley alternatives for the bedridden and, for those who are able, the importance of getting up and around to aid in recovery. For vascular devices, they educate about other less invasive options and ask physicians to critically reassess the need for routine labs given the challenges associated with this process. Patients and families are also given educational materials, such as a one-page explanation of these issues to help them better understand the rationale behind the decisions.

ORGANIZATIONAL CONSTIPATORS

Our use of the word *constipators* is somewhat tongue in cheek, but the term does clinically describe the impact these people—primarily mid- to high-level executives—can have on a quality improvement initiative.[3] And that impact can be considerable, even though the organizational constipators generally have no animus toward the particular works they are gumming up. They are, in effect, disinterested resisters of the initiative, and they come in two basic varieties.

Some of these people simply enjoy exercising their power. At one hospital, for example, the lead quality manager told us that after attending the first day of training for a project to reduce infections, she was forbidden to attend the second day by the chief nurse. No reason was given, and the chief nurse was not opposed to the project. This was the manager's explanation: it was a "control issue." The chief nurse viewed any independent action by an underling as an affront. Another such person might consider any effort to alter the status quo as a threat to his or her power. What distinguishes these kinds of organizational constipators is that their actions are purposeful.

Their counterparts exercise their power by failing to take action. Memos pile up in their inboxes and overload their email accounts. A physician described his chief of staff in this way: "Somebody who will nod their head and say, 'Well, let me think about it.'" He would keep bringing up an idea he had proposed, and the chief of staff wouldn't remember it, so the physician would have to go back into his own email and resend an old message, adding, "Did you ever make a decision on this?" We heard stories of administrators who kept putting off the hiring of replacement nurses or signing off on purchase orders for lab equipment. An infection preventionist told of having a "huge problem" with an executive who "needs to do certain things and he just doesn't do them."

Aside from the direct damage that organizational constipators can do to safety initiatives, they can also lower staff morale and sour professional relationships, both of which are so essential to an initiative's success. The physician quoted previously put it this way: "You just lose energy." A key problem with organizational constipators is that their bosses think they are effective workers, whereas their underlings cannot believe the constipators still have their jobs.

Organizational constipators are more difficult to cope with than active resisters, in part because their negative effect on a quality improvement intervention is a function of their normal operating style. There is no upset over extra work, no quarrel with the science of the bladder bundle, no negative attitude toward a particular nurse champion—attitudes of the active resister that at least lend themselves to being changed. In the case of the organizational constipator, the barrier to a successful intervention is rooted in some basic personality traits.

The managers of initiatives often try to work around these people. At one hospital, where the director of nursing was a notorious roadblock, the project manager told her little about the bladder bundle initiative and went over her head if there was a problem. A quality manager in a similar situation commented, "Basically, if I keep off the radar, I can do what I need." Some hospitals revise their organizational charts so that these troublemakers retain their title, but their responsibilities are reassigned such that they can do less damage.

A potentially more effective strategy was described by a hospital director: "Well, I think if you have a systematic way of addressing major issues through an executive board. . . . Essentially we've brought a particular person who's known for . . . having strong opinions into these discussions and so we are able to vet them." The director explained the hazards of working around these individuals:

> I think so often organizations take that person and keep them out because they're going to block maybe something that you wanted, and we put them over here instead of bringing them into the fold and . . . I've seen that in a couple of specific situations where it's been so helpful to have that person there and have the dialogue, and in a couple of instances, you know, they changed their mind or turned into a supporter of it.[3]

Eventually, though, some institutions run out of patience with organizational constipators. "The tough approach is what we've done here," a chief of medicine told us, "and that is, they're gone." Otherwise, hospitals can wait until such a person leaves or retires. When the opportunity does appear, they need to take their time in finding a replacement to make sure they're not simply trading one problem for another.

TIME-SERVERS

"I don't have a clue what to do with either the stupid or the lazy," the chief of surgery said. "I have no way to make them work better." The people who fit the category we call "time-servers" are more likely to be lazy than stupid. They are essentially serving out their time, doing the least possible for their role and position. Quality improvement initiatives are someone else's problem; they don't stick their necks out for anyone.

Even when a time-server nurse has been fully briefed about, say, the bladder bundle and the importance of removing a Foley in a timely manner, she'll find ways to do nothing. We learned of a nurse who promised her supervisor that she would talk with a doctor about removing a Foley over the weekend. When the supervisor returned on Monday, nothing had been done. Time-servers seldom follow through.

They take the course of least resistance: Do what the doctor says. If the patient wants to keep the Foley in place, don't bother discussing with her the pros and cons of that decision. In fact, keep a Foley in patients as long as possible because it's easier that way. When it comes to intravenous devices, they try to make sure their day-to-day work is not hampered. Removing an idle central line or PICC makes their work harder when it comes to drawing labs or infusing medications. It's easier for them to have the device remain in place.

Short of having them fired, which is often a problem because of union rules, hospitals can try to change the behavior of time-servers by giving them daily reminders of the elements of a safety intervention and having an authority figure frequently reinforce the reminders.

We also favor another, admittedly demanding, approach for coping with time-servers as a group. We have observed that they tend to multiply in institutions burdened by a culture of mediocrity. If the leadership of a hospital is satisfied with second best, the environment will be rife with time-serving. The cure is drastic: a conversion to a culture of excellence. It requires that the hospital instill a devotion to patient-centered, high-quality care in each and every unit, along with the full-bore support of quality improvement initiatives. Eventually, the psychological effect on time-servers would be comparable to what happens when a shopper finds herself in a Whole Foods store without a reusable bag. "She will run back to the car to get a reusable bag," a physician told us, "because people look at you funny in that store if you don't have one." If a unit or a floor of a hospital is dedicated to a patient safety initiative, time-servers who don't shape up will be seen as shirkers and shunned. If that doesn't bring them around, nothing will. We provide (see Box 7.1) an overview of the three types of healthcare workers who bedevil quality interventions along with a summary of some field-tested approaches to cope with them.

In addition, we offer a recap of two new studies that seek to identify the reasons hospitals succeed or fail—at quality improvement in general and at implementing infection prevention initiatives in particular.

WHY HOSPITALS STRUGGLE

While many studies have sought to explain why high-performing health-care organizations succeed, relatively few have tried to understand why so many hospitals are struggling with preventing infections. That deficiency has been addressed in a systematic review[8] of 30 studies of underperforming hospitals—a review undertaken by a team of experts in implementation science, patient safety, and research reviews. By singling out some of the major reasons for these institutions' troubles, the authors hoped to provide fresh targets for quality improvement efforts.

In selecting the 30 studies, the team identified the organizations studied as "struggling" when they had below-average patient outcomes, as reflected in their mortality data or inadequate quality of care, as shown in their Patient Safety Indicators scores. On the other hand, the studies that were chosen for analysis were all qualitative, including interviews, rather than quantitative because important aspects of any institution—its culture, for example—do not lend themselves to understanding via a statistical or numerical approach. The studies included acute care hospitals (13 studies), emergency rooms (one study), nursing homes (three studies), outpatient primary clinics (seven studies), specialty clinics (one study), primary health systems (one study), accountable care organizations (one study), hospital units (two studies), and residential treatment programs (one study).

The team found that these low-performing institutions consistently struggled with five areas: a poor organizational culture; an inadequate

Box 7.1

STYLES OF PERSONNEL BARRIERS[a]

Challenging Staff Styles

1. Active resisters to a change in practice are pervasive, whether the resister is an attending physician, a resident physician, or a nurse. Successful efforts to overcome active resistance include the following:
   a. Data feedback comparing local infection rates to national rates.
   b. Data feedback comparing rates of compliance with the rates of other hospitals in the same area.
   c. Effective championing by an engaged and respected change agent who can speak the language of the staff he or she is guiding (e.g., a surgeon to motivate other surgeons).
   d. Engage the resister's participation in collaborative efforts that generally align hospital leadership and clinicians with the goal of reducing HAI.
2. Organizational constipators—mid- to high-level executives—act as insidious barriers to change in practice. Once leadership recognizes the problem and the negative effect on other staff, various techniques can be used to overcome these barriers.
   a. Include the organizational constipator early in group discussions in order to improve communication and obtain buy-in.
   b. Work around the individual, recognizing that this is likely a shorter term solution.
   c. Terminate the constipator's employment.
   d. Take advantage of turnover opportunities when the constipator leaves the organization by hiring a person who has a very high likelihood of being effective.

3. Time-servers are essentially serving out their time, doing the least
   possible. These staff members are the hardest to overcome. Short of
   firing them, some suggestions include
   a. Provide daily reminders of the elements of the safety
      intervention and have an authority figure frequently reinforce
      the reminders.
   b. Promote a culture of excellence.

ª Adapted from Saint et al.[3]

---

infrastructure; a lack of cohesive mission and vision; planned and unplanned events called "system shocks"; and dysfunctional external
relations.

Poor Organizational Culture

Every struggling organization explored in the 30 studies was found
to have a problematic culture. Staff members' commitment to the
institutions' goals, values, and standards of behavior was limited, at best.
Systems of accountability were fragmented, so that employees consistently sought to avoid responsibility for their decisions and actions, and
generally succeeded, while senior managers tended to stay above the fray.
Employees had little sense of ownership of the enterprise and often felt
ineffective in their work. Failures were frequently blamed on one or another aspect of their patient population—too many of them old and frail,
for example.

Another theme that emerged from the analysis of the 30 studies was a
general absence of collaboration within the culture of the struggling organizations. Because employees felt disconnected from each other and
their institution, their morale was low, and they were more likely to go
their own way instead of working together. Sometimes, patients suffered.
In one case, because two nurse assistants assigned to a unit had failed to

communicate properly, a patient in the unit went without care throughout an eight-hour shift.

The cultures of the low-performing organizations also included a tendency toward a traditional, hierarchical relationship between supervisors and subordinates. An employee in an institution where that relationship was strictly enforced described how supervisors reacted when workers asked for an explanation of a decision: "'Why' is considered a bad word here. They don't want to share the power. If you do [ask], you get shot down. It's that hierarchical thing." In the 30 studies, a rigid hierarchy was often cited by middle managers and quality improvement champions as robbing them of the authority they needed to do their work. It was mentioned by nurses and other staff as a reason they felt undervalued. In some studies, it inspired feelings of anxiety and fear.

A fourth culture-related theme was of a leadership motivated more by the institution's financial concerns than by its mission and the needs of its staff. As a result, the top people were content to set low-quality goals and settle for mediocre results as long as there was no impact on the bottom line. They had little direct communication with their employees. One staff person described his personal connection with his CEO: "I would say minimal, minimal. They had some problems with the previous CEO. And after that, there was an interim guy that I met just once."

Inadequate Infrastructure

Twenty-seven of the 30 studies reported weaknesses in the institutions' basic facilities and operations, and 20 of those studies listed inadequate quality improvement systems as a major infrastructure failing. There was limited use of formal problem-solving tools or an organized collection of performance data.

Weak personnel procedures were another infrastructure-related theme behind the struggles of the low-performing healthcare institutions. The staffing was frequently insufficient, and that problem was particularly noticeable among the nurses. They had a high turnover rate, which led to the use of staff members with less formal training, especially in the surgical ICUs.

There was recognition among all the struggling organizations that information technology was a key to improved quality performance, but they were unable to harness it because of deficient computer facilities, weak computer system management, or both. Often, when they approached information technology for assistance, they would be relegated to the back of the line of improvement requests, derailing their goal of moving forward on a project.

The fourth infrastructure-connected theme was a general absence of resources. The studies mentioned hospitals that simply could not collect timely and accurate data. The resources missing here were just as much manpower as experience. Many hospitals had the right number of people, but they lacked the skill set and technical expertise needed to execute on a project.

Lack of Cohesive Mission and Vision

An organization's mission statement identifies its basic goals and how it plans to achieve them. Its vision statement describes the desired organization of the future. In the case of the low-performance organizations, the mission was poorly defined and the vision cloudy, at best.

A major theme among the institutions studied was the ongoing conflict between their stated missions (patient care) and management's unwritten mission (dedication to the institution's economic viability and regulatory compliance). That left the staff confused by contradictory requirements, disappointed in their personal aspirations, and lacking in the motivation so essential, for example, to an institution's quality improvement efforts.

The staffs of the struggling organizations experienced similar feelings of confusion and disappointment when they realized that their organizations' vision was being defined externally. That happened when their leaders suddenly gave their highest priority to reducing readmissions, this after Medicare announced financial penalties for high readmission rates. The staff's conclusion was that their organization was driven not so much by what was best practice for patients but what was best for the bottom line.

The goals of the low-performing organizations studied were poorly defined. Quality improvement, for example, was often attempted as a kind of graduated effort, with limited goals—say, a "substantial" reduction in the incidence of a disease. Aiming for that kind of general improvement proved to be of limited benefit in inspiring staff buy-in. High-performing hospitals, on the other hand, have success in motivating staff by aiming for an absolute standard of zero in reducing, say, CLABSI.

System Shocks

For many of the struggling institutions, organization-wide events— planned and unplanned—wreaked havoc with day-to-day operations. The events set forth in the studies ranged from frequent changes in the top leadership to the arrival of new technologies to a sudden surge in turnover.

The 30 studies found that many of the low-performance institutions were subject to recurrent shake ups in the C-suite (also known as C-fever). Said a staff member at one of those institutions, "Over the last four years . . . we've had four or five CEOs." Chief executives and their leadership cadre are normally the driving force in any organization, but it takes months, even years, for new top-level personnel to properly fulfill that role. They don't understand the operations and culture of the organization, so, as one study put it, "Sporadic involvement of senior management was common . . . in part because of frequent turnover." The new leaders have an uphill battle earning the support and loyalty of the staff, for as another report found, "An explosive level of turnover made connectivity almost impossible."

Financial failure, or the threat of same, was noted in a quarter of the 30 studies. Such monetary troubles reverberate throughout an institution. Budgets are cut, hiring is halted, and staff members worry about their future and look for new jobs. One of the studies concluded, "We found that widespread concerns about finances . . . eclipsed attention paid to patient safety."

Mergers were among the system shocks that rocked the struggling organizations. One study, for example, spoke of their "fragmented systems of accountability . . . a legacy of recent mergers." Another study reported on the damage to an organization's operations by the in-house conflict that so often occurs when two cultures are merged. A staff member of one of the low-performance institutions likened the situation to the reunification of Germany after the fall of the Berlin Wall.

Sometimes the very efforts to improve quality had a negative impact on the struggling organizations. Major change of any kind can be disruptive. Some studies cited the introduction of a new electronic health record (EHR) as an example. Another example is wide-scale quality improvement programs. As one study noted, "Changes aimed at improving established organizations often caused an initial decrement in their performance as a result of the substantial reorganizations."

Among the system shocks suffered by the struggling institutions were scandals and other public relations crises. A singular instance cited was the waiting list fiasco experienced by some Veterans Affairs hospitals. When a scandal suddenly emerges, it strikes at the morale of the institution's staff members and lowers their efficiency.

Dysfunctional External Relations

Seven of the studies spoke of the hospitals' history of poor connections with key stakeholders. That was true as well of their relationships with local and regional levels of government; in fact, there was little contact at all with key administrators outside the walls of the hospital. And although these struggling institutions claimed that they collaborated with postacute providers, the actual relationship was not well developed.

These characteristics of low-performing healthcare organizations represent clues to an understanding of why they are doing poorly. Such clues, the authors of the systematic review suggested, may provide a "first step" for the low performers as they go about the task of self-improvement.

A EUROPEAN PERSPECTIVE

What helps and what doesn't when hospitals set out to prevent CLABSI? The authors of one study[9] sought to answer that question through an in-depth, qualitative study of CLABSI interventions at six hospitals in different parts of Europe. The six were split between those most likely to succeed and those more likely to fail as a way to highlight the circumstances and strategies that promoted the intervention and those that hindered it.

The study was part of the Prevention of Hospital Infections by Intervention and Training (PROHIBIT) project, financed by the European Commission.[10] The goal of the larger project, as well as the six-hospital study, was to observe and analyze CLABSI interventions based on two scientifically approved approaches—a hand hygiene (HH) program and a comprehensive strategy governing central venous catheter insertions (CVCi's).

Nurses and ICU physicians from all the hospitals taking part in the PROHIBIT project were invited to a two-day workshop for training in the upcoming infection prevention effort. Before the intervention began, investigators spent two days at each of the hospitals and conducted interviews and made observations. They repeated the process a year into the interventions. There were also telephone interviews conducted between those visits. The interviewees ranged from the top management level, to members of the infection prevention team, to all levels of the ICU.

Among the six hospitals included in the study, three implemented both HH and CVCi protocols, two implemented just CVCi, and one only implemented HH. Each hospital developed its own strategy, and they did not always align with PROHIBIT's agenda. That was particularly the case among hospitals in countries with higher healthcare expenditures.

To entice hospitals to join in the study, PROHIBIT had offered each potential participant hospital the services of a half-time nurse, but sometimes these nurses ended up in nonintervention projects. One hospital, for example, which had been randomly assigned to implement the HH program, already had a long history of HH efforts. The infection prevention team there decided to use the nurse to pursue other infection prevention efforts in the ICU, such as ridding it of long-sleeve apparel. Even though there was no significant reduction in their already modest CLABSI rates among the hospitals in countries with higher healthcare expenditures, they perceived the intervention as a success.

Hospitals in countries with lower healthcare expenditures and high CLABSI rates also viewed their interventions as successful, in their case because their CLABSI levels dropped significantly. The half-time nurse was particularly valuable in terms of standardizing procedures. The PROHIBIT training sessions also contributed to the success of the interventions. A nursing director, for example, hailed the "collaboration outside the hospital," noting that a previous implementation at the hospital "was not easy."

All six of the hospitals' interviewees listed limited resources as a factor that handicapped their pursuit of the CLABSI initiative. Even hospitals in countries with higher health spending were affected by economic disruptions: Hiring was halted, and professionals who left hospitals were not replaced. The restrictions were far worse in hospitals in countries with lower health spending. Physicians and nurses routinely held two jobs, stayed on after retirement age, or left for better opportunities. As a hospital CEO recalled, the nurses who left didn't earn any more in their new jobs, but their hours were better. "Like when these supermarkets opened," he said, "then a lot of nurses went there to work."

These conditions sometimes sapped the staff's support of the CLABSI initiative. A head infection prevention physician spoke of nurses who were exhausted from caring for extra patients: "Of course they don't really care about this project. And they have low salaries and are thinking about going abroad." In Eastern Europe in particular, many doctors and nurses had been wooed away by foreign universities and hospital systems. In the process, the local hospitals lost staff members trained in the PROHIBIT protocols as well as nurses responsible for their implementation.

The availability of material resources essential to the implementation was also reduced by budget constraints. Some hospitals were forced to do without alcohol-based chlorhexidine skin antiseptic and other necessary items. At one institution, nurses were cutting back their use of alcohol-based hand rub and gloves in order to lower costs.

Yet there were hospitals that succeeded in marshaling the human and material resources needed to achieve PROHIBIT goals. To a major degree, the six-hospital study found, the distribution of resources was determined by three kinds of change agents: nurse and physician champions within the hospitals; the influence on hospital leadership of having to live up to the standards of a national program; and the impact of disruptive events—a CLABSI outbreak that inspired greater staff participation, for example, or a hospital's entire relocation that prevented implementation.

The human change agents were often what the study authors called "boundary spanners," staff members whose multiple roles helped them bridge built-in institutional barriers and accelerate change. They were generally described by their colleagues as well respected and possessed of "huge knowledge about both intensive care and microbiology or epidemiology," as one interviewee put it. At a hospital said to have a top-down culture, two boundary spanners had joint appointments in the ICU and the infection prevention and control (IPC) program. An ICU/IPC boundary spanner nurse said she was the usual point person for infection prevention projects because "I know the equipment, I know the staff, I know how it's done, and I know the ICU."

At another hospital, the boundary spanner was a former medical director. He used his access to the C-suite to lobby for funds to support the CLABSI intervention. When the CEO signed on, the needed materials were ordered.

Boundary spanning also occurred across informal networks. Nurse and physician champions of the PROHIBIT implementation were able to obtain the cooperation of staff members in their own and other units because of personal relationships. In some cases, the connection was friendship. An ICU physician distinguished between "the people above me that decide" and those "directly connected with me and are friends."

As for the friends, he went on, "It's quite easy to work with them. We go to the restaurant."

Relationships formed at interdisciplinary committee meetings also helped some boundary spanners with the CLABSI project. Staff members from different wards became acquainted at these sessions. So, when a committee member serving as a project champion called on another committee member in a different area for assistance, it wasn't a cold call.

The absence of boundary spanners, the study found, could have a strong negative effect on the PROHIBIT effort. An ICU head nurse, for example, spoke of the powerful hierarchy in her hospital. "There's no way I would go to the nurse director and ask for something," she said. "I would go to the nurse superior, and the superior to his superior, and so on. Everything is too slow. Things are not moving forward."

The study concluded that the ability of a hospital to engage its staff in the PROHIBIT implementation and provide the human and material resources needed for success was most often achieved by means of committed boundary spanners.

In the next chapter, as promised, we describe the collaborative option, the joining of a group of hospitals to pursue a specific quality improvement initiative. It is an alternative to the single-hospital model we have focused on up to this point. Collaboratives have become extremely popular, particularly in efforts to prevent HAI. They may be a good option for some hospitals, but they do have their drawbacks.

SUGGESTIONS FOR FURTHER READING

Krein SL, Damschroder LJ, Kowalski CP, Forman J, Hofer TP, Saint S. The influence of organizational context on quality improvement and patient safety efforts in infection prevention: a multi-center qualitative study. Soc Sci Med. 2010;71:1692–1701.

    In this article, the authors closely examined quality improvement efforts and the implementation of recommended practices to prevent CLABSI in US hospitals. They compared and contrasted the experiences among hospitals to better understand how and why certain hospitals are more successful with practice implementation. Their findings provide important insights about how different quality improvement strategies might function across organizations with differing characteristics.

Krein SL, Kowalski CP, Harrod M, Forman J, Saint S. Barriers to reducing urinary catheter use: a qualitative assessment of a statewide initiative. JAMA Intern Med. 2013;173:881–886.

Krein and colleagues purposefully sampled 12 hospitals that were participating in the Michigan Health and Hospital Association Keystone Center for Patient Safety statewide program to reduce unnecessary use of urinary catheters (the bladder bundle). The authors interviewed key informants to identify ways to enhance CAUTI prevention efforts based on the experiences of these hospitals. In the article, the authors presented barriers to implementation and strategies to address them.

Saint S, Kowalski CP, Banaszak-Holl J, Forman J, Damschroder L, Krein SL. How active resisters and organizational constipators affect health care-acquired infection prevention efforts. Jt Comm J Qual Patient Saf. 2009;35:239–246.

The authors collected qualitative data from phone and in-person interviews with hospital staff from a national study to determine the barriers to implementing evidence-based practices to prevent HAI, with a specific focus on the role played by hospital personnel. They found that, in particular, two types of personnel—active resisters and organizational constipators—impeded infection prevention activities, and that hospital personnel used several approaches to overcome these barriers.

Vaughn VM, Saint S, Krein SL, et al. Characteristics of healthcare organisations struggling to improve quality: results from a systematic review of qualitative studies. BMJ Qual Saf. 2019;28:74–84.

In this systematic review of 30 qualitative studies, five domains characterized struggling healthcare organizations: poor organizational culture (limited ownership, not collaborative, hierarchical, with disconnected leadership); inadequate infrastructure (limited quality improvement, staffing, information technology, or resources); lack of a cohesive mission (mission conflicts with other missions, is externally motivated, poorly defined or promotes mediocrity); system shocks (i.e., events such as leadership turnover, new EHR system, or organizational scandals that detract from daily operations); and dysfunctional external relations with other hospitals, stakeholders, or governing bodies.

Joining a Collaborative

A single arrow is easily broken but not ten in a bundle.
—Japanese Proverb

His hospital, along with dozens of others, had just participated in a quality improvement collaborative, and the infection preventionist was impressed—to a degree. For years, he had tried, and failed, to convince the attending physicians to update their approach to central lines. "If nothing else," he said, "this project has been instrumental in getting that change to happen. Before, it was me fighting the wolves."

Yet the infection preventionist was dissatisfied with the project's overall impact. It had the vocal support of the hospital's top officials, he explained, "but we never got the backing monetarily or time-wise." Even though many staff members wanted to participate, they were not allowed to take time away from their regular duties, so the collaborative became "just another one of those things," as he put it, just another in a long list of demanding quality improvement initiatives.

A similar ambivalence can be found in many studies of collaboratives. Even as this communal approach to enhancing healthcare has been taken up by more and more hospitals across the country and won support from federal agencies and dozens of state governments, questions remain about its effectiveness. There are a variety of collaborative models, but in this chapter we look at the operation of a generic quality improvement collaborative. This is a short-term commitment for each hospital—a 12- to 24-month project focused on a limited number of goals, such as improved outcomes for central line–associated bloodstream infection (CLABSI) or catheter-associated urinary tract infection (CAUTI). This is as opposed to a long-term collaboration of hospitals that work together for years toward a common broader goal, such as improving the quality of care for hospitalized medical,[1] surgical,[2-5] or pediatric[6,7] patients (e.g., through a series of initiatives). We focus on aspects of these short-term collaboratives that differ from the kind of single-hospital initiative described in the previous chapters. And, we suggest how a hospital and its project team can make the most of the collaborative experience.

JAPANESE BEGINNINGS

The history of the quality improvement collaborative can be traced back to the 1980s and the emergence of the continuous improvement process in Japan. As preached by Kaoru Ishikawa and W. Edwards Deming, the continuous improvement process assumes that you can endlessly improve a manufacturing process by continuously gathering and evaluating feedback about how the process is actually working out and then applying what you've learned to improve the process. This program of incremental improvement is central to kaizen, the practice that helped Toyota revolutionize automotive manufacturing worldwide.

The feedback mechanism was eventually adapted to the needs of healthcare with the routine collection and analysis of data about patients and medical outcomes as a path toward better treatment options. That technique is a staple of today's quality improvement collaboratives.

The emergence of the collaborative movement is generally credited to the lackluster quality improvement record of individual hospitals. Pressure had been mounting, from governments and the public, for hospitals to improve their clinical results and to control spiraling costs. The collaborative was seen as a means to both ends, in part by imposing an external discipline on participating institutions. It no doubt also benefited from the universal perception that there is, as Homer put it so many eons ago, "strength in unity."

For example, the French phrase "L'Union fait la force," translated "in unity there is strength" is found on the coat of arms of Haiti and embodies the culture, as exemplified by the Haitian response to the devastating 2010 earthquake.[8] More ominously, the concept was central to the National Fascist Party, which ruled Italy from 1922 to 1943. The party took its name from the Latin word *fascis,* or "bundle," and used a cylinder of birch rods as its symbol; any single rod might easily be broken, but the bundle of rods would endure. By extension, it was hoped that the binding of a number of hospitals into a collaborative would yield a stronger performance than that achieved by individual hospitals. The bundle theory has another application in these pages, of course: The complete set of practices within the bladder bundle has a stronger impact than would those practices implemented separately.

A COLLABORATIVE AT THE MODEL HOSPITAL

Our look at a relatively generic quality improvement collaborative starts early one Monday morning when the chief executive officer (CEO) of our model hospital learns that a national agency is putting together a countrywide collaborative aimed at reducing CAUTI. The model hospital is on its list of intended participants. The CEO asks his top clinical people to consider whether the hospital should take part and eventually calls for a meeting to discuss the matter.

Collaborative sponsors choose their topic with care since it can determine the project's success or failure. The topic needs to be broad enough to appeal to a hospital's administration as important and marketable, yet narrow enough to require no more than a reasonable investment of time and energy on the part of the hospital's staff. It needs to be evidence based and scientific, yet not so technically complicated that it will be difficult to learn. Above all, the topic should require a positive change—but not so much of a change that it will inspire widespread clinical resistance.

At the meeting called by the model hospital's CEO, the chief medical officer—having never read the preceding chapters—reports that the hospital's CAUTI rate is considerably higher than it should be. Both he and the chief nursing executive express concern about the staff time and resources a collaborative would require, especially given the current high number of quality improvement initiatives at the hospital. The CEO acknowledges that argument, but he points out that the sponsoring national agency carries professional and financial clout that can make it difficult for hospitals to ignore an invitation to join the collaborative. In fact, the agency actually supports some of the model hospital's own quality improvement programs. And the CEO recognizes the need to reduce healthcare-associated infection (HAI)—as a medical matter, as a marketing matter now that these statistics are publicly on display, and as a financial imperative since the Centers for Medicare & Medicaid Services stopped reimbursing hospitals for many HAIs. He also doesn't want to be odd man out by refusing to join the collaborative if his peers at nearby hospitals sign on. After weighing all the benefits and challenges, he decides to join the collaborative effort. The CEO asks the chief nurse to take it over.

To serve as the sponsor, leading the model hospital's participation in the collaborative, the chief nurse chooses his or her deputy, the director of nursing—who, in turn, selects as project manager the unit manager of a first-rate inpatient nursing unit. A physician champion and a nurse champion are then recruited, along with the infection preventionist, completing the core membership of the project team. (The core membership of the CAUTI prevention team was discussed in Table 5.1 of Chapter 5.)

Though it takes just a few sentences here, the selection of the team's sponsor, leadership, and composition has actually been a careful and somewhat lengthy process. The chief nurse understands that the intervention is a complex and inherently difficult project, the participants driven by a variety of sometimes conflicting motives. Those devoted to advancing their careers, for example, may be more interested in the chance to meet with clinicians from other hospitals and the leadership title than in the responsibilities that go with that title. The CEO may be more eager to show the hospital's flag than to properly finance the initiative. The chief nurse knows that if the team leaders are not willing to work within the requirements and discipline of the collaborative, the project is doomed from the start.

AN 18-MONTH PROJECT GETS UNDERWAY

At the statewide kickoff meeting, the core team from the model hospital and teams from dozens of other hospitals meet the faculty experts from various professional societies who will be their instructors and mentors during the course of the collaboration. A representative from the sponsoring agency lays out the essentials of the 18-month project: the widespread impact of CAUTI on patients, the scientific evidence behind the bladder bundle, the importance of removing inappropriate Foleys, and, in particular, the need to gain the cooperation of bedside nurses and other front-line staff. They may have good reason to be resistant because of the extra demands of the initiative on their time, especially since there have been several recent in-house quality projects. There will be more educational sessions before the actual intervention begins and regularly scheduled telephone and in-person meetings. The collaborative is designed to maximize these learning interactions—it is an important component of the project's "strength in unity."

In all their early presentations, the experts ask the model hospital and the other participants to plan their initiatives with long-term sustainability in mind. The processes that will be changed during the implementation should be hardwired into the hospital's operations from the get-go: The CAUTI prevention nursing template should be understood to be a permanent addition, for example, and that should be true of the monitoring of Foley rates as well. The project leaders and champions should be selected for the long term: Are they the kind of people who will ensure that the benefits of the initiative will live on once the collaborative has run its course?

Each hospital's project leaders will have to arrange for a baseline assessment of indwelling urinary catheters and the incidence of CAUTI and maintain a daily record of those data throughout the implementation. The baseline data and a monthly update will be shared with the managers of the collaborative. During the planning phase, there will be calls every other week, with extra time devoted to sessions on how to collect, organize, and analyze these data and on processes that have proven to be a major stumbling block for earlier collaborative teams.

During these group calls, experts offer advice and answer questions. In this way, as they exchange ideas, a sense of community forms and a behavioral norm evolves. The educational efforts also include a website with transcripts of the educational sessions and answers to frequently asked questions, as well as regular webinars that feature discussions of the project's basics and of implementation challenges—along with possible solutions—that have come up at several sites.

Once the actual implementation begins, all teams, regardless of how far along they are in the project, are required to take part in two calls each month, one state and one national. The calls are informal and interactive, providing opportunities for teams to share their experiences and help each other overcome problems. Each team is also expected to provide monthly electronic reports of its CAUTI data, keeping the collaborative leadership and other teams aware of everyone's progress—or lack of progress. New strategies are welcome: The project manager at the model hospital, for example, reports on its program to have a nurse trained in the bladder bundle take part in multidisciplinary rounds, keeping an eye out for inappropriate Foleys and urging their removal if found; the program has led to a substantial drop in the rate of Foley use.

Social occasions are designed to build the teams' comfort level, relieving the feeling some team members have that they are alone in this challenging endeavor. The social encounters also build mutual trust, encouraging the teams to share experiences, including best practices. These gatherings occur during the three in-person learning sessions: at the kickoff, at the 9-month midway point, and at the end of the collaborative. Time is set aside during lunch and coffee breaks to allow teams to intermingle and interact. These "constructive collisions" are one of the key rationales for the in-person meetings.

The front-line activity in a quality improvement collaborative is similar to that found in a single-hospital initiative as are many of the problems, including active resisters, organizational constipators, and time-servers. However, there are other potential difficulties that can arise because of the very structure of the collaborative. The team leaders at each hospital have presumably learned a great deal about preventing CAUTI, and in theory, that advice has been effectively communicated to the other members of the project team. In practice, though, that exchange of information is often inadequate. The communication failures occur in the opposite direction, as well, with bedside nurses failing to share the details of their problems with project team members and team members failing to report internal team problems to the project sponsor.

A COOKIE-CUTTER EXPERIENCE

By its very nature, the typical collaborative provides hospitals with a cookie-cutter experience. The educational materials and bladder bundles are identical for all hospitals, the teams track a common set of measures, and participants are expected to follow the same schedules and procedures. Team leaders do have some opportunity to air their particular problems and seek solutions, but, given the collaborative's central direction, there is far less of the natural tailoring of a quality improvement project than can be found in most single-hospital initiatives.

Studies of quality improvement collaboratives have warned about a tendency on the part of organizers to focus on didactic talks, leaving little time for discussions of implementation problems at individual hospitals. Aware of this concern, the experts serving some collaboratives set aside hours for private meetings with teams that are having trouble and have little or no idea why. Some collaboratives have even created a special group, including a physician, nurse, and quality improvement expert, which is available to visit hospitals that are struggling with the implementation process. Usually, the group responds to a request from such hospitals, though it sometimes will volunteer its assistance when a particular intervention is floundering or a hospital appears to be on the verge of dropping out of the collaborative. (By one estimate, up to 30% of hospitals in a collaborative leave the program before its conclusion.[9])

During their site visits, these experts interview a broad cross section of the target hospital's staff—C-suite to bedside nurse—with particular attention paid to the project team members. Gradually, a picture emerges of the hospital's culture, the staff's attitudes toward quality improvement interventions in general, and the roadblocks in the way of this intervention. The experts will then suggest ways to tailor the intervention to fit the local setting. Instead of promoting the bladder bundle as an all-or-nothing proposition, for example, the consultants may propose implementing only those practices that seem feasible given the hospital's context or culture. If the nurse-initiated Foley removal protocol is not tenable, the experts will offer other options (i.e., a computerized reminder for physicians or prominent reminders on patients' charts). If a nurse manager is standing in the way of progress, the expert group will propose ways to bypass the manager. Sometimes a hospital that is unwilling to accept the adaptive aspects of a bundle will be willing to buy a new piece of equipment. Investing in technology is infinitely easier than trying to change individual behavior.

Though the people overseeing the collaborative have no legal power over the laggard hospitals, they do have ways to prod them forward. The various interactions of the teams, built into the collaborative, create a pressure to live up to those teams with the most improved catheter rates. As one physician told us, the collaborative is "a big motivator for us to say, 'OK, we're trying to get ourselves to the same standard as everyone else's standards.'" But that competitive pressure can have a negative impact as well, embarrassing laggard teams. In a study identifying the features that participants in 53 collaboratives found most helpful,[10] one hospital's project manager described the attitude some teams have toward the online interactions: "People just feel intimidated to use it because they don't want to ask a question that people will think is stupid."

The same study found that the sharing aspects of collaboratives such as solicitation of staff ideas and learning session interactions received fairly high ratings. Yet, when the helpfulness of the interactive aspects was broken down between participating teams that improved significantly and those that did not, it showed that interaction received considerably higher helpfulness ratings among the more successful teams. "Our results suggest," the author said, "that collaboratives may work most for participants who capitalize on their interorganizational features in addition to their intraorganizational features."

In some quality improvement collaboratives—such as the Michigan Hospital Medicine Safety Consortium[1] (supported by Blue Cross/Blue Shield of Michigan)—financial incentives are used to spur and implement change. These incentives are performance oriented, with thresholds set based on how the group of hospitals perform on defined metrics. Importantly, the incentives are tiered, such that even incremental change is rewarded with some degree of financial support. To enable quality changes, collaboratives such as the ones in Michigan also provide financial resources for systematic data collection across sites, thus helping hospitals do the important data collection and analysis needed for discovering problem areas and implementing change. For example, in one initiative in Michigan, hospitals systematically collect data on peripherally inserted central catheter (PICC) use and outcomes. A dedicated abstractor at each hospital is partially funded by the collaborative and undergoes rigorous training and assurance to ensure data capture from patients' records is robust. Because they are so close to the data, these individuals often lead data presentations at hospital-wide meetings to point out where individual performance metrics (e.g., use of single-lumen devices or placement of PICCs in patients with chronic kidney disease) may be lower than desired. The presence of the C-suite and hospital leadership at these meetings, often because of the monetary implications of these data, helps ensure that change will have topside support. It is also an opportunity for the project leaders to feel recognized and see the value of their work.

On the face of it, the quality improvement collaborative appears to be a most reasonable approach to the refractory hospital infection problem. Indeed, many studies of collaboratives have reported substantial improvements in infection results, greatly reducing device-associated rates, for example. But systematic reviews of the quality improvement collaborative literature have raised questions, including some about the accuracy of the uncontrolled collaborative studies. As one commentator put it, they "were probably biased in favor of positive findings in successful teams."[11]

The systematic reviews have also found a disturbing lack of consistency in the collaborative outcomes. Why do so many hospitals drop out of collaboratives? Why is the evidence of positive change on the provider level—in terms of medication management, for instance—generally not matched by evidence of comparable gains on the patient level? Why do so many of the hospitals that do well in collaboratives already have a strong, patient-centered, cooperative culture in place and a positive record of successful internal quality improvement initiatives?

THE ADVANTAGES AND DISADVANTAGES OF
A COLLABORATIVE

In general, a collaborative project is of greatest value to hospitals that have the desire to undertake a given quality improvement initiative but lack the tools and the expertise to go it on their own. They don't have to spend their own resources and staff time reinventing the wheel for an in-house quality intervention. Also, collaborative hospitals are often provided instruction for data collection and feedback of data to compare their own performance over time with other hospitals in the collaborative.

A hospital considering a collaborative, however, should be prepared for the inevitable friction that occurs when an outside entity imposes its program on a medical institution. The hospital's clinicians may be told to do things that are against current hospital policy: requiring universal use of alcohol-containing chlorhexidine, for example, or empowering bedside nurses to remove Foleys without physician orders. The record of the hospital's success or failure in meeting the goals of the collaborative, month by month, will be widely broadcast among the participants. And if a hospital taking part in a collaborative does have some expertise in the particular initiative, the hospital should make sure those experts are working cooperatively with the outside experts or the whole project could be put at risk.

Discipline is central to the strength of any collaborative, and participating hospital teams must toe the line if the initiative is to succeed. The teams must perform according to the collaborative leadership's directives. Hospitals that want initiatives that are shaped to fit their particular environment and culture are more likely to prefer running their own, in-house quality improvement projects.

In any event, the lack of a sufficient body of controlled studies of these collaboratives has made it difficult to judge their overall effectiveness. Without such scientific results, the reasons for participants' success or failure in implementing change and the particular aspects of collaboratives that lead teams to move in one or the other direction remain uncertain. Because the collaborative process itself is so complex and varies from one initiative to another, and because the institutions that participate in a collaborative are themselves so infinitely complex, a definitive scientific evaluation of their interaction has remained an unanswered challenge. If possible, the collection of a sufficient quantity of preintervention data is recommended to be able to adequately assess if any reductions seen after the collaborative's initiation are any different from reductions consistent with secular trends, as demonstrated in results published recently from two large collaboratives[12-14] that demonstrated no significant reductions in CLABSI and CAUTI rates compared to secular trends prior to the collaborative.

In the following chapter, our focus turns to the task of sustainability: How can a hospital hold on to the progress it has made during the course of a quality improvement intervention?

SUGGESTIONS FOR FURTHER READING

Fakih MG, George C, Edson BS, Goeschel CA, Saint S. Implementing a national program to reduce catheter-associated urinary tract infection: a quality improvement collaboration of state hospital associations, academic medical centers, professional societies, and governmental agencies. Infect Control Hosp Epidemiol. 2013;34:1048–1054.

In this article, the authors present an overview of the national effort to reduce the risk of CAUTI, funded by the Agency for Healthcare Research and Quality. Based on the successful pilot work in Michigan led by the Michigan Health and Hospital Association Keystone Center, the project has the following key components: (1) centralized coordination of the effort and dissemination of information; (2) data collection based on established definitions and approaches; (3) focused guidance on the technical practices that will prevent CAUTI; (4) emphasis on understanding the socioadaptive aspects; and (5) partnering with specialty organizations and governmental agencies that have expertise in the relevant subject area.

Meddings J, Greene MT, Ratz D, et al. Multistate programme to reduce catheter-associated infections in intensive care units with elevated infection rates. BMJ Qual Saf. 2020;29:418–429.

In a large collaborative of intensive care units recruited for elevated baseline rates of CAUTI or CLABSI, an externally facilitated program intervention was implemented by a national project team and state hospital associations. On-demand video modules and live webinars were among the techniques used in the two-tiered effort to prevent catheter infections, focusing on both technical and socioadaptive factors. The principles and tools of the intervention were based on the Comprehensive Unit-Based Safety Program. Using data from the first two cohorts of this collaborative, and relying on multilevel negative binomial models, the authors found no significant changes in CLABSI, CAUTI, or catheter utilization compared to secular trends.

Nembhard IM. Learning and improving in quality improvement collaboratives: which collaborative features do participants value most? Health Serv Res. 2009;44:359–378.

Using surveys and semistructured interviews, the author identified features that participants in various collaborations supported by the Institute for Healthcare Improvement found most helpful for advancing improvement efforts overall and knowledge acquisition in particular. Nembhard's findings identified features of collaborative design and implementation that participants viewed as most helpful, including interorganizational features.

Saint S, Greene MT, Kowalski CP, Watson SR, Hofer TP, Krein SL. Preventing catheter-associated urinary tract infection in the United States: a national comparative study. JAMA Intern Med. 2013;173:874–879.

In this study, the authors conducted a survey of 470 infection preventionists to compare the use of specific infection prevention practices by US hospitals. Their results showed that Michigan hospitals, compared with hospitals in the rest of the United States, more frequently participated in collaboratives to reduce HAIs (94% vs. 67%), which may have contributed to the fact that Michigan hospitals had a 25% reduction in the rate of CAUTIs (compared to 6% reduction in the rest of the United States).

Swaminathan L, Flanders S, Rogers M, et al. Improving PICC use and outcomes in hospitalised patients: an interrupted time series study using MAGIC criteria. BMJ Qual Saf. 2018;27:271–278.

In this 10-hospital statewide collaborative, a multimodal intervention (including tools, training, electronic changes, education) to reduce inappropriate PICC use and reduce PICC-associated complications was implemented and evaluated in a quasi-experimental, interrupted-time series of one intervention hospital and nine contemporaneous external controls. After adjusting for underlying trends and patient characteristics, however, a marginally significant 14% decrease in inappropriate PICC use occurred at the study site with no change observed at control sites. The incidence of all PICC complications decreased to a greater extent at the study site, but the absolute difference between controls and intervention was small.

Toward Sustainability

> We are what we repeatedly do. Excellence then, is not an act, but
> a habit.
>
> —ARISTOTLE

"Nobody's going to sit back and be comfortable," the infection preventionist
insisted. Her 500-bed suburban hospital had just completed a successful
intervention to reduce its central line–associated bloodstream infection
(CLABSI) rate, but she and her colleagues were not resting on their laurels.
"You're going to push one another to go to that next level," she told us, "because having value and feeling like you make a difference is what makes
you happy in your work."

In the quality improvement field, the ability to sustain and even improve a successful initiative is the holy grail, Ahab's white whale. Various
managerial studies have suggested that up to 70% of organizational
change efforts simply don't survive. Once an initiative stops being an institutional focus, once an organization moves on to other projects, there's
a natural tendency to revert to old ways. The damage may be substantial
when a bank's change program lacks legs, but the demise of a hospital's
quality improvement project—to reduce a healthcare-associated infection, for example—can have dire consequences for hundreds or thousands
of patients.

For all the research about program sustainability, there is no valid, tested formula for doing it right. That's because the institutions and units involved are different from each other in so many ways, including their personnel, their policies, their use of champions, and their culture, not to mention the resources they are willing to commit to any given project. No single set of procedures fits them all. Yet there is a body of best practices that can help a hospital hold on to its quality improvement gains.

THE IMPORTANCE OF EARLY PLANNING

At our model hospital, the institution-wide intervention to prevent catheter-associated urinary tract infection (CAUTI) has run its 18-month course. Foley usage has been cut dramatically, leading to a sustained 30% to 35% CAUTI reduction throughout the hospital. A month before the intervention's end, the original leaders of the project team meet with the executive sponsor to review their work together and discuss what lies ahead: maintaining the progress to date. They know that hospitals too often jump from one change process to another without consolidating their advances. They know that even among institutions that recognize the importance of early planning for sustainability, too many give it lip service and nothing more.

In the model hospital, sustainability was on the agenda from the start. The leaders of the initial intervention were carefully chosen with an eye to their staying power, and team members accepted their posts with the understanding that it would be an ongoing commitment. When the initiative scaled up, that same commitment was made by the new champions in the emergency department, the intensive care units (ICUs), the operating rooms, and the individual floor units. The time requirements would be heaviest during the intervention phase, of course, but everyone knew that they would be needed after the formal initiative ended as well. They also knew that their participation would continue to boost their annual staff evaluation.

At the prevention team's meeting, participants ask themselves how well the hospital is positioned to hold on to its CAUTI prevention gains. To what degree have the mandates of the bladder bundle become institution-alized? Do the physicians and nurses automatically resist inserting Foleys that fail to meet appropriateness criteria? Do they remove Foleys when the catheters are no longer needed?

The team members happily agree that the basic elements of the bladder bundle have, in fact, become routine practice at the hospital. This will make their task much simpler. The director of acute care at a hospital described the sustainability of a CAUTI prevention initiative in her hospital in down-to-earth terms: "It's an everyday thing that we roll with."

Another advantage the team recognizes is their hospital's continuing culture of excellence. Just as it set the table for a successful CAUTI prevention intervention, the shared commitment to excellence underpins the sustainability of this and any such quality initiative.

THE PROJECT TEAM'S ROLES IN SUSTAINING IMPROVEMENTS IN CAUTI AND CLABSI

At the project team's meeting, the leaders agree that the lines of communication between them and the champions in different parts of the hospital must be maintained. The champions remain responsible for keeping an eye on their units, making sure there is no falling off in adherence to the bladder bundle, and alerting the project leaders to problems or potential problems. If one or another nurse or physician champion is about to be reassigned or plans to leave the hospital, for example, his or her replacement must be brought up to speed. In fact, the executive sponsor suggests that the team should routinely urge current champions to develop potential replacements for themselves.

The champions throughout the hospital will also be responsible for providing the infection prevention department with a once-a-week count of the Foleys in their units, a substantial easing of the daily catheter patrol that operated during the intervention. And each month, the infection preventionists will issue a report providing the current and past Foley prevalence and CAUTI rate for each of the hospital's units. It will be sent to all of the units as well as the hospital's administrative and clinical leadership and will be posted on the hospital's website.

Of course, there will always be backsliders, those who revert to the old ways of doing things. A nurse shared with us her problem with a handful of physicians who had always, she said, thought along the lines of, "This patient is incontinent—of course they need a catheter" or "This person is a hard-stick—of course they need a PICC [peripherally inserted central catheter]." She defined her challenge in these terms: "It is changing their paradigm and making it stick. I can think I have them all headed in the right direction and then, six months later, I am back saying, 'Hey, what do you think about taking this catheter out or not placing a PICC in this patient?' with the same physician."

The updated data will enable the members of each unit to measure their progress in the war on CAUTI. Because they are on the front line of that struggle, and because the patients are so directly in their care, these reports are of particular concern to the nurses and nurse managers in the various departments. The intervention has succeeded in large measure because of their acceptance of the bladder bundle changes, and they have a professional and personal stake in preserving that achievement. Any report of an increase in Foley use or in the CAUTI rate is likely to spur them to take corrective action. It's their duty, yes, but it's also a matter of professional pride.

The monthly reports serve another purpose. They remind management that the CAUTI initiative carries on, albeit at a reduced level. That helps maintain C-suite support for the sustainability program and its personnel. It's never a good idea to allow your project to fall completely off the radar screen.

The leaders of the sustainability program at the model hospital are keenly aware of the inevitable arrival of new quality improvement projects and of the time and resources these newcomers demand of clinicians— time and resources that might be stolen from the CAUTI prevention mission. Quality campaigns are so thick on the ground these days that they end up competing against each other. The members of the team are determined that their project will not be viewed as part of that competition.

They want it to be seen as providing benefits for other safety efforts, as a potential partner in new interventions.

If a quality initiative to reduce pressure ulcers appears at the hospital, for instance, the CAUTI prevention team will link to it, pointing out that Foleys tend to keep patients immobile and more susceptible to the ulcers. Thus, both the pressure ulcer and CAUTI projects share the goal of using Foleys only when medically necessary and removing them as soon as possible. The CAUTI prevention effort can also be linked to the Surgical Care Improvement Project, which focuses on significantly reducing surgical complications. Because the absence of a Foley in postoperative patients allows for their greater mobility, it can also promote more rapid recovery. Finally, because many critically ill patients have both Foley catheters and central lines and are at risk for both CAUTI and CLABSI, focusing efforts within and beyond the ICU to link resources for addressing both goals is often important for these complex patients.

One challenge to the sustainability of the CAUTI prevention initiative, as suggested above, will be the arrival of new physicians and nurses at the hospital, people who may not be familiar with the requirements of the bladder bundle. To prepare for this, the team leaders will make sure that online CAUTI prevention instruction and other educational materials are part of the hospital's orientation process, and they assure each unit champion that they stand ready to help if there are problems with any newcomers. The director of a medical ICU who was sustaining a CLABSI prevention initiative described the orientation process: "That's like an on-going thing. . . . People coming in from hospitals across the country who aren't doing this. They're learning a whole new system, so it's kind of intense training. Everybody up to speed all the time."

That process is somewhat eased by the fact that the new arrivals are often younger and more open to fresh ideas than their predecessors. "It is hard to teach an old dog new tricks," an infection preventionist told us with some satisfaction, "but with a new puppy it is easy."

Openness to change, the project leaders recognize, should also apply to the postintervention period as a whole. Sustainability should not equal entrenchment. The champions should always be alert to any possible improvements that can be made to the ways they support and promote the initiative. Should the Foley data be gathered more often—or less often? Is there a better way to remind bedside nurses of the availability of alternatives to the Foley? Is the patient education material doing the job?

Such questions are on the agenda at the monthly sustainability meetings of the model hospital's project leaders. They also review the latest data from the infection prevention department, looking for changes in Foley prevalence. And they take up any problems that have arisen since the previous session and discuss possible solutions. Yes, the items in the bladder bundle have become second nature for most of the model hospital's clinicians, but there are always a few backsliders to keep track of and a few newcomers to watch out for—and the need to help one or another unit champion find a replacement. At a meeting of the leaders of a quality improvement project committed to sustaining change, there's always something to talk about.

The experience at one hospital is instructive. An intervention there reduced the number of inappropriate catheters to nearly zero—and cut CAUTI rates by 39%.[1] To sustain these advances, the hospital continued to use, as part of routine nursing care, a computerized nursing template for assessing which patients on each shift had a catheter and whether that catheter met appropriateness criteria. If the catheter was considered inappropriate, it would be removed. As part of the effort to hardwire the intervention, physicians received a monthly email message from the chief of medicine to remind them that CAUTI prevention continued to be a priority and to reiterate his support for having the nurses essentially be stewards of the urinary catheters. The name of the physician champion was displayed in the email in case other physicians had questions. Finally, monitoring of important outcomes, such as the proportion of catheters that were appropriate and the CAUTI rates, continued. These data were shared with the front-line staff as well as with others in the organization. The results of this approach were impressive: Three years after the CAUTI prevention initiative began, the hospital recorded a 12-month period with just a single CAUTI.

In another sustainability study,[2] this one following up on Michigan's Keystone ICU intervention, the much reduced rates of CLABSI at the end of the intervention were maintained and even further reduced after 18 months. During interviews at the participating hospitals, ICU team members pointed to the continuous feedback of infection data and the active involvement and support of senior leadership as major contributors to sustainability. The feedback provided the team with a kind of report card on their efforts, alerting them to any increase in infection or offering proof that CLABSI was still under control.

An important gap in preventing CLABSI that is necessary for sustainability is how best to prevent infections that result from inappropriate catheter care and maintenance. Insertion of a central line only accounts for a tiny share of its total life—yet, the majority of interventions to prevent CLABSI have been targeted to the insertion. Thus, four maintenance best practices have been the focus of recent studies: (1) hand hygiene before accessing the catheter; (2) scrubbing the catheter hub with an alcohol-containing product for at least 15 seconds followed by 15 seconds of drying time before accessing the lumen; (3) ensuring integrity of the dressing by performing daily inspections and prompt assessment of wet, loose, or soiled dressings; and (4) removing unnecessary or idle catheters as soon as clinically possible. Studies that have examined permutations and combinations of these approaches have shown promising results, especially in preventing CLABSI beyond seven days of catheter dwell, when most infections are thought to be the result of inappropriate catheter handling. Hospitals have developed protocols that emphasize these process measures during daily nursing huddles and rounds. For example, at the University of Michigan, data on catheter care are collected and presented at the system CLABSI steering committee on a monthly basis and reported by unit level, such that deviations from best practice can be investigated and understood. Additionally, new technologies to ensure that the catheter entry site or the hubs of the catheter are protected from bacteria (e.g., chlorhexidine-impregnated sponge dressings or alcohol caps) are potential escalation strategies to consider when compliance to these measures is ensured. In this manner, sustainability of a CLABSI initiative and expansion to include care and maintenance with ongoing data evaluation can be achieved. This model of continuous improvement is explored in future chapters as well.

MAINTAINING PROGRESS IN HAND HYGIENE

Among the most urgent sustainability goals, in general, is the effort to maintain progress in improving hospitals' hand hygiene practices. Perhaps the single most important cause of healthcare-associated infection is the widespread failure of healthcare workers to follow proper handwashing procedures. Some hospitals are successful with sustained improvements, such as a successful hand hygiene intervention that increased rates from 18% to 32.5%, which was sustained (31.9%) at five years after an initial contest-based intervention in three Japanese hospitals.[3] Intervention sustainability can vary between healthcare workers at the same institution because of differences in leadership.

We authors have also participated in hand hygiene sustainability studies at hospital units in Florence, Italy, where we saw how an intervention's substantial progress in improving hand hygiene could be sustained over a four-year period in one unit—and how another unit's adherence to the handwashing protocol plummeted after the hand hygiene champion left his leadership post.[4] In the unit with stable leadership, adherence held at 71% compared to 37% before the intervention began. In the unit that lost its champion, adherence dropped among nurses from 51% to 8%. Among physicians, the fall was from 51% to 3%! An active leadership and team effort are key elements in sustaining any quality improvement. Similarly, after initial improvements in hand hygiene in two infectious disease units in an Italian hospital, reassessment of hand hygiene after a change in leadership that occurred because of a merger demonstrated that improvements in physician hand hygiene persisted (from 51% to 63%) in the setting of a persistent physician champion for hand hygiene, though nurse hand hygiene fell significantly from 36% to 24% with the lack of a nurse champion after the merger.[5]

Thus far in the book, we have focused on examples of hospital infections that arise from the use of devices. But as we noted in Chapter 1, our approach to gaining the cooperation of clinicians in the adoption of preventive interventions can serve as a model for other important hospital initiatives, such as preventing other hospital-acquired infections or complications such as pressure ulcers or falls. In the next chapter, we show how the principles illustrated for developing and implementing successful CAUTI prevention programs can be applied to an initiative aimed at preventing *Clostridioides difficile* infection, an increasingly common hazard of hospitalization.

SUGGESTIONS FOR FURTHER READING

di Martino P, Ban KM, Bartoloni A, Fowler KE, Saint S, Mannelli F. Assessing the sustainability of hand hygiene adherence prior to patient contact in the emergency department: a 1-year postintervention evaluation. Am J Infect Control. 2011;39:14–18.

In this study, the authors assessed the sustainability of a previously published, successful hand hygiene intervention in a pediatric emergency department in Florence, Italy. They found that compliance one year after the initiative (~45%) was consistent with that immediately postintervention (~45%). Their data also showed that there was an increase in adherence over this time among nurses (41% to 50%) and a marked decrease among physicians (50% to 36%). These results indicate the differences that can develop between healthcare providers during a sustainability program.

Fakih MG, Rey JE, Pena ME, Szpunar S, Saravolatz LD. Sustained reductions in urinary catheter use over 5 years: bedside nurses view themselves responsible for evaluation of catheter necessity. Am J Infect Control. 2013;41:236–239.

In this study of non-ICUs at an 800-bed tertiary-care teaching hospital in Michigan, the authors evaluated the effect of a multimodal intervention to increase appropriate urinary catheter use and the ability to sustain that compliance. During the five years of the study, there was a significant reduction in urinary catheter use, from 17% to 13% ($p < .0001$).

Lieber SR, Mantengoli E, Saint S, et al. The effect of leadership on hand hygiene: assessing hand hygiene adherence prior to patient contact in 2 infectious disease units in Tuscany. Infect Control Hosp Epidemiol. 2014;35:313–316.

In this study of an infectious disease unit at a hospital in Florence, Italy, Lieber and colleagues assessed the sustainability of a successful multimodal hand hygiene initiative over four years. They found that hand hygiene adherence among all healthcare workers was significantly higher four years after the intervention (71%) compared with preintervention rates (37%). A study of another infectious disease unit that had not participated in the intervention but was under the direction of the intervention's physician champion demonstrated a significant drop in adherence among nurses (51% to 8%) and among physicians (51% to 3%) after he retired. The results of this study illustrate the success of the intervention as well as the effects of leadership on hand hygiene practices.

Stirman SW, Kimberly J, Cook N, Calloway A, Castro F, Charns M. The sustainability of new programs and innovations: a review of the empirical literature and recommendations for future research. Implement Sci. 2012;7:17.

In this review of the research literature, the authors evaluated 125 studies related to sustainability. They found that most published studies were retrospective, and approximately half relied on self-reported data. They were equally divided between quantitative and qualitative methods, and few of them employed rigorous methods of evaluation. Research in this area is lacking in respect to the extent, nature, and the impact of adaptations to the interventions or programs once implemented. The results of this search suggest that while prospective and experimental designs are needed, there is also an important role for qualitative research in efforts to understand the phenomenon, refine hypotheses, and develop strategies to promote sustainment.

Taking on *Clostridioides difficile*

All diseases begin in the gut.

—Hippocrates

In 1893, pseudomembranous colitis was first described in a surgical patient being cared for by the surgeon John Finney and Sir William Osler.[1] At the time, no one knew the cause of this novel gastrointestinal finding, but over the years it became a frequently encountered complication of antibiotic use and was even referred to as "clindamycin colitis." Researchers set out to gain a better understanding of this disease, and in the 1970s it was realized that it was a result of an infection with *Clostridioides* (previously called *Clostridium*) *difficile* in the colon.[2,3] When these early researchers studied *C. difficile* infections (CDIs) in rodents, they noticed an interesting curiosity. When the hamsters were housed in a new facility that had never accommodated subjects with CDI, they had to intentionally feed *C. difficile* bacteria to the rodents to induce the disease; however, in well-established animal facilities, direct introduction of *C. difficile* into the diet was not necessary; the rodents seemed to spontaneously develop the infection from the environment itself.[4] That same result occurs in human facilities as well: Hospitals all too often function as a nidus of infection for CDI.

In the decades since this realization, hospitals searched for effective ways to control *C. difficile*, yet its incidence has soared as new, more virulent strains have emerged. For reasons both technical and socioadaptive, hospital initiatives to cope with *C. difficile* have frequently fallen short. There is a lack of randomized, gold standard studies to support a number of the current best practices used to prevent and control the infection, which has led some hospital personnel to oppose quality interventions based on those practices. The *C. difficile* prevention bundle also requires difficult behavioral changes. In fact, though *C. difficile* and catheter-associated urinary tract infection (CAUTI) are very different, the adaptive aspects are similar in many ways. In this chapter, we show how the adaptive approach of the previous chapters on CAUTI can be applied to *C. difficile* prevention.

THE NATURE OF *C. DIFFICILE*

The *C. difficile* bacterium exists in both a metabolically active vegetative form and in the form of a dormant spore that can survive for months or even years without nutrition. It is fairly common and has been found in water, vegetables, animals, and even soil. However, exposure to the *C. difficile* bacterium does not always lead to infection. Both toxigenic and nontoxigenic varieties exist, and small-scale colonization in the gut usually produces no symptoms. It is the exposure to a large number of toxigenic strains in the right clinical setting that leads to an infection. These types of exposures are widely associated with contact with the healthcare system. The infection—producing abdominal pain, fever, intestinal inflammation, and diarrhea—generally strikes those who have a weakened defense system and are not able to fend off the pathogen. These are the elderly, the infirm, and people with an abnormal intestinal microbiota. And once a person has the infection, the chance of a recurrence can be as high as 20%.

Infection with *C. difficile* is a major public health problem. The Centers for Disease Control and Prevention (CDC) actively monitors this infection and estimates that 223,900 cases of CDI occurred in 2017 in hospitalized patients in the United States, which resulted in at least

12,800 deaths.[5] While community-onset CDI does occur, studies indicated that an exposure to the healthcare environment is usually associated with new infections. Given this, there have been many efforts by healthcare systems focused on developing and implementing strategies to prevent CDI.

When the administrative and medical leaders at our model 250-bed hospital decide to pursue a *C. difficile* initiative, they are responding to some of the same pressures they faced with their CAUTI initiative. The hospital's infection rate is too high, increasing the risk for patients, but there are marketing and financial concerns as well. Since 2013, hospitals must publicly report CDI rates to the Centers for Medicare & Medicaid Services for all to see. Then, in 2015, CDI joined CAUTI on the list of healthcare-associated infections (HAIs) that are no longer eligible as a diagnosis that could increase hospital payment by CMS when acquired in the acute care setting. This is no small cost, as each infection with *C. difficile* increases the average hospital stay by 2.8 to 5.5 days and costs hospitals an estimated $3,006 to $15,397.[6] Given the increased safety, improved public image, and cost savings, the decision to support a CDI prevention program is an easy one.

ASSEMBLING THE TEAM

Once the C-suite has agreed to undertake a *C. difficile* prevention program along the CAUTI and central line–associated bloodstream infection (CLABSI) lines, the next step is to create the team. As with the CAUTI and CLABSI initiatives, the members of the team will depend on the different aspects of care that play a role in CDI. The model hospital's *C. difficile* prevention team has a multidisciplinary makeup, including someone from senior leadership, a project manager, physician and nurse champions, an infection preventionist, and laboratory personnel. But there are also some important early additions to the team, including a manager from environmental services to coordinate room cleaning and an inpatient pharmacist, who will be a key figure in antimicrobial stewardship.

One of the team's first decisions concerns the scope of the intervention. The CAUTI project team chose to follow the path of caution, testing and improving a pilot initiative before scaling up. But, there are compelling reasons for the *C. difficile* prevention team to start big. Many elements of *C. difficile* prevention—special room-cleaning directions and antimicrobial stewardship, for example—can be more efficiently and effectively implemented on a full-scale basis.

KEY APPROACHES TO CDI PREVENTION

Now that the team and scope have been determined, the team has to decide what interventions to implement in addressing three large goals in the fight against CDI: preserving patients' defense against infection, preventing their exposure to the bacterium, and improving the diagnosis of the disease.

Defensive Measures

The patient's best defense against CDI is a robust intestinal microbiota. The number of bacteria in the normal human intestine is higher than the number of cells in the rest of the body. These bacteria are a diverse group, representing over 1,000 different species that live in a delicate balance so that no one species is over- or underrepresented. When patients are exposed to antimicrobials, this balance gets significantly disrupted, creating an opportunity for *C. difficile* to take hold and proliferate. In this way, the use of broad-spectrum antimicrobials increases a person's chance of developing CDI by 7 to 10 times while taking the drugs and for a month thereafter.[7] Often, these antibiotic exposures are entirely appropriate and necessary to treat life-threatening infections, but there are exceptions. In a study at a nursing home in Rhode Island, more than 40% of the patients were found to have been given antimicrobials unnecessarily.[8] Based on a recent meta-analysis of 11 studies, hospitals that implemented an antimicrobial stewardship program saw a 32% cut in CDI.[9] Despite their importance, antimicrobial restrictions do not always sit well with physicians and nurses—or with patients and their families, as we shall see (see Box 10.1).

Antimicrobial stewardship is a quality initiative unto itself, addressing a range of issues not limited to *C. difficile* prevention. The project team at the model hospital examines the current policies for prescribing antimicrobials—and finds it wanting. The hospital epidemiologist and pharmacist design a new protocol that restricts the use of high-risk, broad-spectrum antimicrobials (e.g., levofloxacin), requiring preapproval of their prescription except in emergent cases. The protocol receives the appropriate endorsements and is then widely distributed within the hospital, supported by occasional educational sessions held over the course of the intervention.

The team also considers other options and finally decides to include an improvement in the management of all antimicrobials in the intervention. Clinical pharmacists begin reviewing the charts of patients on any antibiotics to determine whether the drug, dose, and duration are appropriate. If, based on the indication, culture data, and other clinical data, the antibiotic prescribed is inappropriate, the pharmacist will contact the prescribing physician to discuss the matter. Should the issue not be resolved, the hospital epidemiologist (who is also an infectious disease physician) is asked to weigh in.

Protective Measures

The model hospital's *C. difficile* prevention bundle also emphasizes the need for protective measures to halt exposure to *C. difficile* bacteria in the acute care setting. Recognizing that patients infected with *C. difficile* widely shed spores and bacteria in their diarrhea, the team develops interventions to limit this contamination. The primary culprits for contamination are the healthcare environment, shared patient equipment, and healthcare workers' hands and attire. Patients with CDI must be identified

Box 10.1

BARRIERS TO ANTIMICROBIAL STEWARDSHIP[a]

Like many drugs, antimicrobials have the potential to both benefit and harm the patient for whom they are prescribed. Unique to antimicrobials, however, is the potential to harm others because of the spread of *C. difficile*. Moreover, excessive widespread use of antimicrobials has also created a host of deadly antimicrobial-resistant bacteria within the general population. Thus, prescribing antimicrobials for a patient with a possible bacterial infection—who may or may not benefit from their use—requires a physician to weigh the potential benefit for the patient against the potential harm to the patient and society.[11] This long-standing tension is a manifestation, at least in part, of an even longer standing battle played out between the political philosophies of John Locke and Jean-Jacques Rousseau.

As one of the authors noted in an essay in *JAMA Internal Medicine*,[10] Locke—a 17th-century British physician whose theories influenced America's founding fathers—believed in the importance of the individual as "free and equal" and in the individual's right to make decisions based on his own judgment and beliefs. In order to best protect themselves and their property, individuals form a body politic, thereby agreeing to certain standards of behavior. Self-interest leads people to form governments; however, individuals may dissolve their government if it ceases to work solely in their best interest. In short, government has no sovereignty of its own.

Jean-Jacques Rousseau, an influential 18th-century European philosopher, argued that the "general will"—a collectively held will that prioritizes the common interest—is far more important than individual will. Writing in *The Social Contract*, Rousseau argued: "whoever refuses to obey the general will shall be compelled to do so by the whole body. This means nothing less than that he will be forced to be free."[12]

The tension between advantaging society or the individual plays out daily when physicians decide whether to prescribe antimicrobials in the hospital. More often than not, the interest of the individual prevails, and antimicrobials are prescribed. This, in part, reflects a very strong desire on the part of clinicians to avoid the chagrin associated with withholding antimicrobials in a patient ultimately found to have a bacterial infection. So, in these daily battles, the emphasis on individualism espoused by Locke appears to rule the day. As a result, there has been little progress in reducing antimicrobial overuse.

ᵃAdapted from Flanders and Saint.[10]

---

early and placed in isolation; they are, ideally, housed in private rooms with private bathrooms or, at a minimum, put with other CDI patients. Patient equipment will not be shared, and, whenever possible, disposable equipment will be used. After patients depart, their rooms are to be decontaminated with a "sporicidal" solution, such as bleach, which has been proven effective in killing *C. difficile* spores. Full barrier precautions, including gloves and gowns for all clinicians caring for the patient, are required. In particular, meticulous use of gloves as well as hand hygiene after glove removal is required given studies holding that neither soap and water nor alcohol-based hand rubs are particularly effective at removing *C. difficile* spores.[13-15]

Diagnostic Stewardship

Balancing the need for early diagnosis, isolation, and treatment is the need for a correct diagnosis of CDI. That process is complicated by the fact that a diagnostic test may be positive for a patient who is not infected but is actually only asymptomatically colonized. Such unnecessary testing can artificially raise rates of CDI and consume scarce resources. All test data must be judged alongside the patient's clinical picture: Is she suffering from diarrhea? Is there another likely cause for her diarrhea (e.g., laxatives, oral contrast, or tube feeds)? Is she currently, or has she, recently been on antimicrobials?

The model hospital has empowered nurses, trained in the process, to speed up the identification by sending a watery stool to the lab for testing without waiting for a physician order. As well, appropriateness measures for when to reject tests for *C. difficile* are provided to lab technicians so that testing is not done on formed stool samples, so-called "stool stewardship." Clinicians are alerted in instances of inappropriate use of testing, such as repeating tests and sending tests to assess for cure. The team also wants to look into the type of testing used by the laboratory. While nucleic acid amplification tests such as polymerase chain reaction are highly sensitive and specific for determining the presence of toxigenic *C. difficile*, they can lead to overdiagnosis if they are not paired with strong stool stewardship or are not used in a multistep diagnostic algorithm.

SUPPORTING THE CDI QUALITY IMPROVEMENT PROJECT

Just as the urinary tract infection rate is collected at the start of a CAUTI initiative, the hospital's precise CDI rate preintervention will be measured as a baseline, and it will be monitored regularly throughout the project. Before the actual intervention begins, the project manager arranges for the education of the team members and the hospital as a whole about the risk factors for CDI, the ways in which it spreads, and the way it is diagnosed and treated as well as the elements of the planned prevention bundle. Both in-person and online educational approaches are used. There are several meetings at which the responsibilities of the various team members are discussed and front-line workers given the opportunity to ask questions and fine-tune the plan.

The team members are also alerted to some of the barriers that clinicians and staff members might encounter. Like the CAUTI intervention resisters, the project manager warns there will be staff members who simply find the proposed changes inconvenient. People from environmental services, for example, may object to using sporicidal cleansers because of the unpleasant odor. Physicians may accept some items better supported by evidence but question the less well supported mandates. Some of them will surely bristle at having their antimicrobial prescriptions second-guessed. In general, doctors don't like to be told how to practice medicine.

The bundle provides a checklist of requirements for preventing *C. difficile*, and once the actual intervention begins, the project manager sees to it that a copy of that list is widely available. Reminders are issued for those clinicians who resist, and posters listing the relevant parts of the bundle are placed in prominent locations in all of the hospital's clinical areas (see Table 10.1).

Patients and their families are informed about the infection and the initiative, seeking their cooperation in preventing its occurrence and its spread. They are encouraged to speak up if a nurse or physician fails to obey any of the bundle's injunctions. They are also asked not to lean on their physician to prescribe a broad-spectrum antimicrobial because it can so easily bring on CDI.

The good communications among the members of the project team, established before the start of the intervention, make it possible to cope with the inevitable unexpected problems. The project manager appeals to the executive sponsor for fresh funds to satisfy the sudden demand for supplies such as gloves and gowns and to provide overtime pay for the understaffed environmental services crew, now facing extra cleaning demands. Nurses appeal to the physician champion to have a heart-to-heart talk with an attending physician who regularly neglects to wash her hands with soap and water after examining a patient with *C. difficile*, instead relying on the alcohol-based hand rub that she routinely uses with other patients.

The infection preventionist on the team makes sure that the surveillance data are regularly dispatched to the team members, the hospital administration, and the various clinical units, where it serves as a goad to improve participation in the intervention and as evidence of progress in combating the infection.

Once their stool is normal, patients are typically released from the hospital while still on antimicrobial therapy to treat the CDI. At the model

Table 10.1 Clostridioides difficile Infection (CDI) Checklist[A]

Hospital Interventions to Decrease the Incidence and Mortality of Healthcare-Associated C. difficile Infections

Prevention Checklist	Treatment Checklist
When an MD, PA, NP, or RN suspects a patient has CDI: Pt has new onset diarrhea (>3 unformed stools within 24 hours) without an alternative explanation (laxatives, tube feeds, oral contrast)	*When an MD, PA, or NP diagnoses initial non-fulminant CDI:* All of the following criteria are present: new-onset diarrhea (>3 unformed stools within 24 hours), no ileus, no bowel obstruction or perforation, no toxic megacolon, no peritoneal signs, and no evidence of septic shock
Physician, Physician Assistant, or Nurse Practitioner: • Initiate Contact Precautions Plus • Order appropriate stool C. difficile testing • Discontinue nonessential antimicrobials • Discontinue antiperistaltic medications • Avoid PPI without strong indication	*Physician, Physician Assistant, or Nurse Practitioner:* • Initiate oral vancomycin 125 mg 4 times daily for 10 days • If no clinical improvement by 5 days after treatment, consider FMT • If true vancomycin allergy (not "red man syndrome"), then use fidaxomicin 200 mg by mouth twice daily for 10 days
Registered Nurse: • Obtain unformed stool sample for C. diff diagnostic test • Place patient in single-patient room • Place Contact Precautions Plus sign on patient's door • Ensure that gloves and gowns are easily accessible from patient's room • Place dedicated stethoscope and other appropriate patient equipment in room • Remind staff to wash hands with soap and water following patient contact	

Prevention Checklist	Treatment Checklist
Microbiology Laboratory Staff Person:	*When an MD, PA, or NP diagnoses initial fulminant CDI:* At least
• Reject formed stool samples inappropriately sent for *C. difficile*	one of the following criteria is present: hypotension or septic shock,
testing, informing relevant clinicians	ileus, bowel obstruction, toxic megacolon, bowel perforation, or
• Inform relevant clinicians of positive *C. difficile* toxin test result	peritoneal signs
• Provide list of positive test results for Infection Control	*Physician, Physician Assistant, or Nurse Practitioner:*
Infection Control Practitioner:	• Initiate oral vancomycin at dose of 500 mg every 6 hours
• Monitor microbiology results daily for positive *C. difficile* test	• Initiate metronidazole 500 mg IV every 8 hours
results	• Minimum duration of treatment 14 days, potentially longer
• Confirm that patients with evidence for CDI are under	depending on clinical course
appropriate isolation precautions (single-patient room with the	• If ileus or bowel obstruction, add vancomycin 500 mg in 500 mL
Contact Precautions Plus sign on the door)	by retention enema every 6 hours
• Investigate root causes for all hospital-onset CDIs (>48 hours	• Strongly consider infectious diseases consultation
after admission)	• Consider obtaining abdominal CT scan
• Alert housekeeping that the patient is on *Contact Precautions Plus*	• Strongly consider surgical consultation to assess need for
	potential colectomy

(*continued*)

Table 10.1 Continued

Prevention Checklist	Treatment Checklist
Environmental Services Staff Person: • Prior to discharge cleaning, check for *Contact Precautions Plus* sign on the patient's door • If *Contact Precautions Plus* sign is on the door, clean high-contact areas in the room with a sporicidal cleaning agent such as a bleach-containing solution • Confirm with supervisor on need for terminal deep cleaning of *Contact Precautions Plus* rooms	*When an MD, PA, or NP diagnoses a recurrent CDI: recurrence is defined as repeated symptoms (after initial resolution) and positive testing ≤ 8 weeks from the start of the original episode* *Physician, Physician Assistant, or Nurse Practitioner:* *First Nonfulminant Recurrence:* • Consider infectious diseases consultation • Initiate oral vancomycin 125 mg four times daily for 14 days then taper over 5–11 weeks • If vancomycin taper cannot be performed, then initiate oral fidaxomicin 200 mg twice daily for 10 days *Second Nonfulminant Recurrence:* • Strongly consider infectious disease consultation • Initiate oral vancomycin 125 mg four times daily for 14 days, then taper over 5–11 weeks *For all fulminant recurrences:* • Strongly consider infectious disease consultation • Strongly consider surgical consultation • Repeat primary therapy, then taper over 5–11 weeks • Consider FMT

Abbreviations: BM, bowel movement; CT, computed tomography; FMT, fecal microbiota transplant; IV, intravenous; MD, medical doctor; NP, nurse practitioner; PA, physician assistant; PPI, proton pump inhibitor; RN, registered nurse; WBC, white blood cell count.

ª Adapted from McDonald et al.[16]

hospital, prior to discharge, these patients are counseled to continue following the bundle directions at home, washing hands with soap and water, and using a separate bathroom cleansed with bleach.

Throughout the intervention, the team leaders are alert to special circumstances that may require adjustments to elements of the bundle, either because of the nature of the patient population, for example, or because one or another element conflicts with established hospital policy. The CAUTI-type approach leaves room for interventions to be tailored to the particular needs or concerns of the individual hospital.

NEW TREATMENT DEVELOPMENTS

As a result of changing epidemiology and resistance patterns that emerged in recent decades, the Infectious Disease Society of America (IDSA) and Society for Healthcare Epidemiology of America (SHEA) recently updated their clinical guidelines for CDI.[16] Metronidazole was no longer recommended as a first-line treatment for nonfulminant CDI since several studies showed that it had inferior treatment response to oral vancomycin. Additionally, the previous severity criteria were simplified and now only distinguish between fulminant and nonfulminant CDI, as detailed in Table 10.1.

A number of new treatments for CDI have recently become available. Among them, the procedure known as fecal microbiota transplant (FMT) has attracted the most public attention. It involves the transfer of donor feces in patients with recurrent or nonresponsive CDI in order to replenish the protective microbiota. This practice has become so widespread that there are several nonprofit stool banks. While several studies support the efficacy of FMT, it does come with risks, as some immunocompromised adults who received FMT developed invasive infections caused by multidrug-resistant pathogens that were present in the donated stool.[17] Researchers have also successfully developed monoclonal antibodies to the *C. difficile* toxins, such as bezlotoxumab, which has been approved for treatment to prevent a recurrence of the infection.[18] Immunotherapy may eventually lead the way to a vaccine to prevent CDI among patients who are at high risk.

In the following section, we examine some of the new approaches, both technical and adaptive, that are being explored in the effort to reduce hospital infections. Meanwhile, though, too many hospital interventions to combat CDI in particular and HAI in general are achieving only modest results today. We believe that the adaptive approach described in this and previous chapters, and in the STRIVE (States Targeting Reduction in Infections Via Engagement) intervention described below, can be applied to a substantial range of medical conditions to significantly improve those results.

NEW APPROACHES TO CDI PREVENTION

In a single year, *C. difficile* was responsible for close to a half-million infections in the United Sates, and some 29,000 people died within 30 days after diagnosis. In acute care institutions, *C. difficile* is the number one cause of HAI. Between 2001 and 2010, for example, its incidence among hospitalized patients soared from 4.5 to 8.2 cases per 1,000 adult discharges, and it has remained at that level despite dozens of major interventions.[19] To make matters worse, a new strain of *C. difficile* has emerged in populations that have not been in a hospital or been given antibiotics—a strain that appears to be more resistant to antibiotics.

Similar to CAUTI and CLABSI, the STRIVE collaborative approach to combatting CDI echoed the two-tier model used with CAUTI and CLABSI, with the Guide to Patient Safety (GPS) serving as struggling hospitals' pathway from the basic strategies of Tier 1 to the enhanced practices of Tier 2. In the appendices, we share a two-tier approach (Appendix C, Figure C.3) and GPS (Appendix D, Box D.3) for prioritizing CDI prevention interventions for implementation. But CDI is a very different kind of infection from CAUTI and CLABSI, as are the means by which it can be prevented, detected, and treated.

The single most important item on STRIVE's Tier 1 agenda for the *C. difficile* intervention was to establish an antibiotic stewardship program

(ASP). There is evidence that ASP implementation is associated with a 32%–52% reduction in CDI incidence.[19] This CDI reduction results not only from gut microbiota preservation, but also from a potentially decreased shedding of *C. difficile* spores. ASPs also have other benefits, such as cost reduction and prevention of multidrug-resistant organisms.

Tier 1 next called for strong stewardship for the diagnosis of CDI. This diagnosis not only has to be early, but also has to be appropriate and accurate. Given high rates of *C. difficile* colonization, clinically significant diarrhea without another etiology should be identified before proceeding to lab tests. The use of a multistep approach using both enzyme immunoassay and nucleic acid amplification tests was recommended. The education of healthcare personnel in the life cycle and epidemiology of CDI was suggested as well.

Recognizing the need to limit exposures to *C. difficile* spores, Tier 1 recommended that the staff of the hospitals participating in STRIVE take precautions in their contact with CDI patients—including the use of protective gowns and gloves in any encounter. Neither alcohol-based hand rubs nor soap and water are particularly effective in removing *C. difficile* spores, so the donning of gloves when entering a patient's room was urged. Special care was suggested in putting on and removing gowns and gloves to avoid contamination. Since medical equipment, such as a rectal thermometer or a stethoscope, can so easily become contaminated with CDI, the use of dedicated or single-use equipment was urged. The use of single rooms or cohorting patients with CDI in the same room was also emphasized. Appropriate environmental cleaning and disinfection can reduce a room's contamination and thus the risk of CDI transmission and infection. Tier 1 called on hospital staff to work with environmental services to make sure that patients' high-touch surfaces (e.g., bedside tables and commodes) as well as healthcare workers' high-touch surfaces (e.g., doorknobs and computers) were targeted.

The STRIVE hospitals were also urged to monitor and share their CDI prevention performance data. These data can help focus interventions on those hospital areas with high CDI rates. If shared with front-line staff, it can also motivate them to participate more enthusiastically in the CDI intervention.

Tier 2 is designed for hospitals whose high *C. difficile* rate had not been appreciably lowered by following the Tier 1 recommendations. They were asked to answer the questions posed by the CDI GPS, and their responses triggered a set of enhanced strategies and resources to help overcome barriers. For example, if a hospital's answers indicated that their lab was not rejecting formed stools that had been submitted for CDI testing, the *C. difficile* GPS would direct the hospital to links where best practices for such a problem could be found.

Among the enhanced practices recommended in Tier 2 is that hospitals begin full contact precautions as soon as lab tests are ordered for a symptomatic patient—and continue those precautions until the patient has been discharged. Such a practice can sap a hospital's human and material resources, but it underscores the fact that CDI patients often remain asymptomatic *C. difficile* carriers even after their diarrhea stops.

Another Tier 2 strategy calls for an intensified focus on environmental cleaning and disinfection. It suggests such interventions as the use of sporicidal cleansers and no-touch disinfectants—ultraviolet germicidal irradiation, for example. Another recommendation is fluorescent markers to make sure that high-contact areas have been properly cleaned.

Tier 2 also suggests approaches to help staff follow the above practices, including team rounding and audit checklists. In addition, greater emphasis is placed on providing staff with real-time feedback on their hospital's adherence to the CDI prevention strategies.

When the results[20] were in, 38% of the STRIVE hospitals had a reduction of 30% or more in the CDI rate. Overall, there was a statistically significant decline in CDI incidence from 7.0 to 5.7 cases per 10,000 patient-days. However, these declines were consistent with temporal trends and could not be definitively attributed to the study intervention.

SUGGESTIONS FOR FURTHER READING

Bagdasarian N, Rao K, Malani PN. Diagnosis and treatment of *Clostridium difficile* in adults: a systematic review. JAMA. 2015;313:398–408.

This systematic review focuses on the clinical diagnosis of CDI. Various diagnostic modalities are discussed in detail, and a diagnostic algorithm is provided.

Dubberke ER, Carling P, Carrico R, et al. Strategies to prevent *Clostridium difficile* infections in acute care hospitals: 2014 update. Infect Control Hosp Epidemiol. 2014;35(suppl 2):S48–S65.

In this compendium, the authors highlighted some of the practical recommendations for acute care hospitals in their efforts to prevent CDI. Strategies for CDI identification, prevention, and treatment are reviewed in a concise format and using available evidence.

Dubberke ER, Rohde JM, Saint S, et al. Quantitative results of a national intervention to prevent *Clostridioides difficile* infection: a pre-post observational study. Ann Intern Med. 2019;171:S52–S8.

In this supplement, the authors described a prospective, quality improvement program across multiple hospitals and states funded by the CDC to reduce infections in acute care settings. Additional detail is provided for the development of *C. difficile* specific interventions, including the Guide to Patient Safety.

McDonald LC, Gerding DN, Johnson S, et al. Clinical practice guidelines for *Clostridium difficile* infection in adults and children: 2017 update by the Infectious Diseases Society of America (IDSA) and Society for Healthcare Epidemiology of America (SHEA). Clin Infect Dis. 2018;66:987–994.

These are updated clinical guidelines on the prevention, diagnosis, and treatment of *C. difficile* put out by IDSA and the SHEA. These thorough guidelines also included a systematic weighing of the quality of the evidence and the strength of the recommendations.

Rohde JM, Jones K, Padron N, Olmsted RN, Chopra V, Dubberke ER. A tiered approach for preventing *Clostridioides difficile* infection. Ann Intern Med. 2019;171:S45–S51.

This article, as part of the STRIVE supplement, outlines a stepped approach for the prevention of CDI. Tier 1 approaches prioritize interventions that are strongly supported by evidence and are less burdensome, such as preventing exposure to *C. difficile* spores, and improving diagnostic stewardship. Tier 2 approaches tend to be more intensive interventions with greater costs, such as performance of a CDI needs assessment and implementation of new environmental cleaning processes.

The Future of Infection Prevention

I hate predictions, especially about the future.

—Yogi Berra

The future of the struggle to prevent healthcare-associated infection (HAI), like its present, has two major ingredients—the adaptive and the technical. In this chapter we discuss both, though, as in the previous chapters, our emphasis is on the adaptive, behavioral change.

To our delight, several so-called future strategies discussed in the previous edition of this book have since been realized. These include the development of the web-based and open access Guide for Patient Safety tools[1] for four hospital-acquired infections: catheter-associated urinary tract infection (CAUTI), central line–associated bloodstream infection (CLABSI), and *Clostridioides difficile* infection (CDI), as well as methicillin-resistant *Staphylococcus aureus* (MRSA) bacteremia. Other realized preventive strategies discussed in the previous edition include the more common use of antimicrobial coatings of vascular catheters for longer anticipated durations (they are on proffer in the CLABSI Tier 2 intervention) as well as chlorhexidine vascular catheter dressings (they are discussed in Chapter 4).[2-4] Unfortunately, there remains no effective antimicrobial urinary catheter at this time to reliably prevent CAUTI. Despite earlier studies[5,6] that appeared promising, a large randomized controlled trial[7] of two types of antimicrobial urinary catheters—silver alloy–coated catheters and nitrofural-impregnated catheters—disappointed.

The use of biomarkers such as procalcitonin as additional diagnostic tools to distinguish bacterial versus viral etiologies of community-acquired pneumonia—as well as guide discontinuation of antibiotics to improve antimicrobial stewardship—is now fairly common. However, the value of procalcitonin is not yet as clear for improving diagnosis and management of other infections, such as urinary tract infection and chronic obstructive pulmonary disease exacerbations.[8]

Another advancement in infection prevention since the prior edition has been the development and implementation of interventions[9] in the nursing home setting to reduce catheter use and urinary tract infections, as well as to improve stewardship of urinary diagnostic tests and antimicrobials[10] across several clinical settings: acute care, ambulatory care, and long-term care. Impressive success was noted in several recent studies involving nursing home patients, including a recent large nursing home collaborative[11] using a multimodal intervention that yielded a 54% reduction in CAUTI as well as a 15% reduction in urine culture ordering.

BEYOND THE HOSPITAL: KEEPING PATIENTS OUT OF HOSPITALS

One reasonable response to the increase in infections acquired in hospitals, of course, is to keep chronically ill, infection-susceptible patients out of hospitals. The Centers for Medicare & Medicaid Services addressed that goal in 2012 when it began trimming payments to hospitals whose readmission rates for patients with a heart attack, congestive heart failure, or pneumonia were higher than predicted. Growing numbers of hospitals and insurers are arranging for many of these patients to be cared for in their own homes, known as "hospital-at-home" interventions.[12,13] Physicians and nurses visit patients daily, either in person or virtually by telemedicine. When necessary, a variety of diagnostic and treatment options are available in the home, from x-rays and echocardiograms, to oxygen therapy and intravenous antibiotics. One study that compared the cost of treating similar patients at home and in a hospital reported that home care was 19% less expensive with equal or better outcomes.[14]

The COVID-19 pandemic led to intense stresses on acute care hospital bed capacity, which in turn created a major concern for the spread of infection to other patients and to healthcare workers while personal protective equipment was in short supply. Many healthcare systems rapidly developed and implemented telemedicine and home monitoring of pulse oximetry, ambulation, medication compliance, and blood pressure of COVID-19 patients. These systems functioned as an alternative to admission to the hospital for patients who were stable enough to avoid admission or for patients who had improved enough to be able to complete their recovery at home, spending less time in the hospital.

BEYOND INFECTIOUS HARMS: MOTIVATING LESS CATHETER USE BY FOCUSING ON NONINFECTIOUS COMPLICATIONS

It has long been recognized that one of the significant challenges in getting clinicians to focus on the avoidance and removal of urinary catheters is their perception of CAUTI as a low-risk complication. Clinicians also cling to the advantages of catheters, including reliable, convenient urinary volume measurement; dry skin; and a reduction in the hours spent caring for incontinent patients. However, several recent studies[15-17] showed that urinary catheters are associated with common and important noninfectious complications, such as pain, hematuria, the potential of permanent urethral injury from catheter trauma, as well as the impact on sexual function for patients outside the hospital with chronic catheterization. For clinicians and patients, these complications may change the perceived benefit-to-risk assessment of a routine catheterization when an alternative exists, even if less convenient. Therefore, new approaches to prevent CAUTI may be more successful if they provide patient education, clinician education and training, and interventions to reduce iatrogenic noninfectious injury from urethral catheter placement.[18]

BEYOND THE CURRENT DEVICES: TECHNICAL ADVANCES

We'd like to turn now to some of the latest technical approaches and theories intended to prevent hospital infections. The Society for Healthcare Epidemiology of America (SHEA), for example, has proposed a new-look future for hospital clinicians' attire as a means to reduce the role of clothing in the spread of infection.[19] Its guidelines call for nonsurgical staff to be "bare below the elbows," wearing short sleeves, and for the eschewing of wristwatch, jewelry, and neckties during clinical practice as these items can become contaminated with antimicrobial-resistant bacteria. In hospitals wedded to the traditional, long-sleeved, white coat, hooks would be placed at appropriate locations so that the coats could be hung before a clinician had direct contact with a patient. More studies have been published assessing how patient expectations for physician attire may vary by clinical specialty[20-22] and by patient and physician characteristics, including age and gender. For example, patients (especially older patient populations[20]) often prefer a white coat and formal attire as it contributes to feelings of confidence in their provider.[21] However, studies in intensive care and emergency settings often showed that patients preferred physicians to wear scrubs.[20] There still remain differences of opinion on which physician attire will yield better outcomes for patients (e.g., lower infection rates) given limited studies, such as if white coats and longer sleeve lengths are associated with significantly increased infections.[19]

Given disappointing results from prior antimicrobial urinary catheters,[7] one highly discussed method is the use of new technical approaches to reduce the development of biofilm and CAUTIs. In addition to continuing work on other types of antimicrobial catheters, there are efforts to develop nonfouling technologies that focus on prevention or the reduction of biofilm development.[23]

An additional reason for the popularity of the coated devices may be the simplicity of their application—the easy switch of uncoated for coated. And our investigations of quality improvement initiatives suggest yet a third possible explanation. Some hospitals gladly pay the extra cost of the devices, seeking to substitute a technical fix for the adaptive challenges of a quality initiative. The problem is that, by themselves, the devices cannot bring about the changed behaviors necessary to prevent most hospital infections.

Copper has powerful antimicrobial properties; copper-coated surfaces have been proven to cut the presence of bacteria by 99.9% in two hours. In one hospital study,[24] copper surfaces substantially reduced the contamination on frequently touched items such as door push plates and tap handles. Another study,[25] in an outpatient clinic, revealed a halo effect: Copper trays and arms fitted to a phlebotomy chair not only showed a 90% microbial reduction compared to noncopper trays and arms, but also reduced the contamination on their cloth-surfaced chairs by 70%. What has kept hospitals from embracing copper? Primarily, this is its high cost relative to other materials. And despite copper's proven antimicrobial power, clinical data have not shown a reduced risk in HAI: Just because it kills bacteria on the surface, does not mean that it will lead to lower infections in humans. There is a third limiting factor: Because its antimicrobial effect takes a while, copper-coated surfaces are not so effective on toilet seats or other such surfaces where contamination takes place too frequently or too heavily.[24]

The increased focus on infection prevention has inspired a spurt of invention in the field of environmental disinfection, especially given the growing scientific consensus that the hospital environment plays a significant role in the transmission of antimicrobial-resistant bacteria. New devices include robots that emit ultraviolet rays and various implements that pump cleansing gases or vapors into a room. The gases have become increasingly common in acute care hospitals, including where hydrogen peroxide vapor and other processes have been used to sterilize precious N95 respirator masks for reuse during the novel coronavirus SARS-2 (COVID-19) pandemic.[26] Tests of a Canadian system that releases a vapor composed of ozone and hydrogen peroxide in a sealed room[27] have achieved a 100% microbial kill rate in several hospital rooms contaminated with MRSA. The vapor formula echoes nature: The human immune system generates an ozone–hydrogen peroxide mix to combat germs.

One relatively simple type of technical device could have an adaptive impact in infection prevention: electronic tools that improve the physician's awareness that a patient has a central line or urinary catheter in place. Some prototypes of these tools have been developed and evaluated at the University of Michigan. One technology calls for all temporary devices inserted in a patient to carry a microchip, which would communicate with a series of three lights—green, yellow, and red—set above every hospital bed. The microchip would be set according to the particular patient's requirements. If a patient's Foley should be withdrawn within 24 hours, the green light would shine until the 24-hour period was drawing to a close, when the yellow light would shine; finally, the red light would take over. Each microchip would have its own frequency so that, if a patient had two catheters (a Foley and a central venous catheter, for example), there would be two sets of lights and no crossing of signals. The premise behind the device is that physicians and nurses might bypass directions on a patient's chart or even a reminder on their pagers, but they would have a hard time ignoring those lights shining in their eyes. A similar reminder system provides a visual, bedside reminder to physicians to prompt catheter removal. The Patient Safety Display shows the location, duration, and clinical indication for a central line or urinary catheter. It was recently piloted in a medical–surgical step-down unit at the University of Michigan, and clinicians found it helpful, but it was not associated with a statistically significant reduction in catheter use in this small pilot study.[28]

COMBATING DRUG-RESISTANT MICROBES

Much of today's infection prevention effort on the technical side is inevitably focused on drug-resistant bacteria like MRSA and carbapenem-resistant *Enterobacteriaceae* (CRE) because infections caused by these bacteria are becoming increasingly difficult to treat with currently available antibiotics. Another recent emerging multidrug-resistant threat is the fungus *Candida auris*, which can also be challenging for many healthcare facilities to identify using standard culturing techniques.[29] For example, researchers are developing new niche antimicrobials that specifically target patients with antimicrobial-resistant infections. Supporters are calling for the federal government to provide extra financial support and to create a limited approval pathway for these drugs, shortcutting the traditionally large and lengthy clinical trials.

Monoclonal antibodies are laboratory-produced antibodies designed to destroy disease cells without damaging healthy tissue. They have long since been used to treat cancer and rheumatoid arthritis and to prevent transplant rejection; the market was valued at approximately $108 billion in 2017 and by the end of 2023 is expected to generate revenue of around $218 billion.[30] Now, scientists are exploring the use of these man-made antibodies to fight drug-resistant infections, including MRSA and CRE. Some monoclonal antibodies have successfully hindered the growth of *S. aureus*, encouraging the immune system to destroy the bacteria with phagocytes (cells that ingest foreign particles and debris). Molecules necessary to the survival of the drug-resistant bacteria are being attacked by other monoclonal antibodies, a strategy that makes it less likely that the bacteria will be able to mutate to withstand new antibiotics. One group of researchers has developed an antibody vaccine aimed at preventing MRSA from eroding bone around an orthopedic implant; the vaccine targets a protein necessary for bacterial growth.[31]

Yet other drugs are being tested that bypass the bacteria themselves, seeking to lessen the body's response to bacterial infection or deny the bacteria access to the body's resources. Healthy bacteria in the skin have been found to be the body's first line of defense against MRSA. Therefore, some scientists are investigating whether oral doses of probiotics, live micro-organisms including some bacteria that may have health benefits, will reduce *S. aureus* nasal and gastrointestinal colonization. Probiotics are also being looked at as a treatment for CRE.

Scientists are testing faster and more accurate ways to diagnose infections, advances that may help clinicians better judge when and whether to use antibiotics. Instead of relying only on direct clinical symptoms, some researchers are measuring biomarkers released by the body in response to infection. High concentrations of serum procalcitonin, for example, may signal infection, including life-threatening urosepsis. In one study,[32] every member of a group of patients with a high procalcitonin level was shown to have severe bacterial urosepsis, a far more rapid diagnosis than by traditional means.

Researchers have suggested a new reason to cut back the use of antibiotics. Their studies have led them to suspect that the same antibiotics that have been so successful in increasing the growth of livestock and poultry may have the same effect on humans. Perhaps, they say, antibiotics may be partly responsible for the epidemic of obesity in the United States.[33]

New drug delivery systems that obviate the need for catheters and ventilators may play a key role in the future prevention of infections. Nanomedicine, for example, may make it possible to release antibiotics precisely at an infection site deep within the body. Nanomachines have already proven capable of clamping interior arteries and tying sutures in animal studies.

PATIENTS AND PROVIDERS: A CHANGING RELATIONSHIP

Some of the most important and challenging aspects of healthcare's future, including the future of infection prevention, will revolve around the relationship between patients and their healthcare providers. It has long been a relationship of "unequals," with nurses and especially physicians holding the upper hand. That has been particularly evident in the hospital setting, where patients tend to be even more vulnerable and dependent. As diagnosis and treatment options have expanded with the new technology and patients have gained increased access to medical information, the relationship has begun to change. Patients are taking control of their own health in corporate wellness programs, learning from TV medical shows, and researching health issues on the Internet. In some health systems with electronic medical records, patients have electronic access to their own health records and can communicate directly with their physicians. Important health discussions are taking place around water coolers and in schools and community centers. At the same time, public agencies and medical organizations are calling for more of a partnership between doctor and patient—for patient empowerment.

To some extent, what we're seeing today is a confirmation of the theories of Geert Hofstede, a Dutch social psychologist. He studied the ways in which nations differ according to a group of values that include masculinity versus femininity and indulgence versus restraint. One of the values was the willingness of a country's less powerful citizens to accept the existing distribution of power, the status quo. On Hofstede's so-called Power Distance Index, Russia scored 93, indicating a high degree of acceptance, whereas Great Britain, Switzerland, Australia, the United States, and Canada had scores between 35 and 40. Citizens of the lower ranking countries, Hofstede said, "strive to equalize the distribution of power."

American physicians who do infection prevention work in countries high on the Power Distance Index such as Japan soon become aware of the difference between their patients' attitudes toward medical authority and the attitudes of their US patients. Studies show that in the United States today, both patients and healthcare providers favor greater patient and family participation in their own treatment. Both parties believe that increased patient participation can improve hospital safety and bring about better medical results in general. But studies also show that both parties tend to place limits on that participation.

It's one thing for physicians to explain the various treatment options to their patients, but few physicians are willing to have patients make the final treatment decision. We saw in previous chapters how hospital patients and their families can complicate caregivers' efforts to have unnecessary Foleys removed, insisting that the convenience of the indwelling catheter is more important than the risk of infection it represents and the delay in surgical rehabilitation it can cause. Patients are not equipped by training or experience to take control over their medical treatment. In fact, research indicates that they have no burning desire to do so.

More and more patients do want to be informed about the various aspects of their diagnosis and treatment. Many of them are willing to become more active in monitoring both their own physical condition and the hospital care they receive. But they tend to back away from empowerment when it calls for them to decide among treatment options or to confront their providers. In some studies, patients were urged to ask caregivers about to have direct contact with them, "Did you wash your hands?" Most patients had trouble complying. One study[34] found that when a group of hospital patients was willing to confront caregivers, it paid dividends—a 50% increase in handwashing. That was an important result, given all the studies that documented high rates of healthcare worker hand colonization.[35] In that case, all the participating patients felt able to put the question to nurses, but just 35% asked it of doctors. Recent studies have shown that the patients' hands are also an important source of microbial colonization[36,37] that could impact the development of nosocomial infections. Interventions are under study that would assess whether programs to prompt patients to perform hand hygiene regularly while in the hospital or in a postacute care setting would reduce the development of nosocomial colonization or infection.

The patient empowerment movement is a relatively new phenomenon with substantial momentum. In the future, we suspect, hospital patients will become more aggressive on their own behalf, and physicians and nurses will become more comfortable with patients who ask a lot of questions and don't hesitate to express their opinions. We also expect that more clinical providers will move beyond a standardized approach, devoting extra time and effort to understanding and treating each patient as a singular individual with his or her own particular needs.

A variety of public and private agencies and organizations have adopted the patient empowerment cause. The Choosing Wisely campaign is a relatively recent example. Originally conceived by the National Physicians Alliance, it has been taken up by the American Board of Internal Medicine Foundation, and joined by Consumer Reports. The following material is how the organization describes its campaign goal.

Choosing Wisely aims to promote conversations between physicians and patients by helping patients choose care that is:

- Supported by evidence
- Not duplicative of other tests or procedures already received
- Free from harm
- Truly necessary

The campaign asked national organizations representing every major medical specialty for a list of five common tests or procedures that "physicians and patients should question." We see it as no accident that the very first item in the adult Hospital Medicine list reads, in part, "Don't place, or leave in place, urinary catheters for incontinence or convenience or monitoring of output for noncritically ill patients." The Society of General Internal Medicine added a list of its own to the Choosing Wisely initiative with five commonly ordered but not always necessary tests or procedures. The fifth item in the list may also strike a familiar note: "Don't place, or leave in place, peripherally inserted central catheters for patient or provider convenience." These lists are being widely distributed and promoted across the country, and Consumer Reports is creating its own set of patient-friendly materials, all in the effort to help patients prepare for their conversations with caregivers.

There is also a need to prep clinicians. In their interactions with patients, as in the other aspects of their lives, today's physicians and nurses are too often on autopilot, their minds preoccupied with thoughts of decisions to be made, calls to be returned, or an uncertain diagnosis. That kind of mental multitasking is a universal trait, of course, but in recent years it has been on the rise among hospital care providers, in part because of unrelenting and ever-increasing job pressures. One study[38] found that 46% of US physicians reported at least one symptom of burnout. Clinicians are sometimes listening to patients with half an ear, thinking of one thing while doing another, reacting rather than responding.

THE POTENTIAL OF MINDFULNESS

To relieve the stress and get off autopilot, a growing number of healthcare providers are practicing mindfulness, the ability to be totally present and attentive in their lives and in their encounters with patients. The approach has its roots in Buddhist meditation, and its focus is on the processes of the mind. Its modern, secular incarnation, a blend of the teachings of yoga and Buddhism, was developed in part by Jon Kabat-Zinn, a molecular biologist by training, who is the founding executive director of the Center for Mindfulness in Medicine, Health Care, and Society at the University of Massachusetts Medical School. His mindful meditation classes are taught at medical centers around the world.

In these classes, clinicians learn how to achieve a beginner's mind, seeing everything, and every patient, as though for the first time, afresh. They learn how to observe themselves in the moment: Are they taking into account the whole context of the visit to a patient? Are they giving the patient a full chance to describe his or her symptoms and feelings? Are they fully attentive to the needs of the particular patient, undistracted by other thoughts and concerns and unstuck from the rut of their own expertise?

The few existing studies of the efficacy of mindfulness in a medical setting have reported generally positive results. One such article[39] called for a group of physicians, nurse practitioners, and physician assistants to take a standardized written test gauging their level of mindfulness. They were then audio-recorded in encounters with patients, and the patients were later asked to rate the clinicians on the encounters. Those with high scores for mindfulness were more likely to have a patient-centered pattern of communication and a more positive emotional tone; they also received higher satisfaction ratings from their patients.

A major barrier to the widespread adoption of mindfulness by clinicians is time: Classes typically range from a week to a full day once a week for eight weeks. However, another study[40] of physicians who had taken an abbreviated mindfulness class—one weekend and two evening sessions—turned up similar results. The doctors were less anxious and depressed, and they remained so almost a year later.

To better understand the impact of brief mindfulness training in the healthcare setting, we conducted a systematic review of the literature about its effect on the well-being and behavior of hospital providers.[41] Nine of the 14 studies we examined showed significant improvements in the providers' well-being, reducing their stress and anxiety levels and improving their resiliency. Burnout symptoms decreased. None of the studies, however, found that the brief mindfulness training had affected the providers' behavior, clinical or otherwise.

Still, some aspects of mindfulness have been applied to improve patient safety and clinical practice. Present-moment awareness, for example, has been used in the primary care setting, and mindful control of cognitive biases has been suggested as a means to cut back diagnostic mistakes. We have developed a conceptual approach that we call mindful, evidence-based practice. We believe that the mindful focus on clinicians' thinking processes may be helpful in implementing infection prevention initiatives, and we have designed a model (Figure 11.1) to illustrate that concept.

In the model, mindful practice is shown as a cognitive process that moves from the clinician's individual values and experience through awareness of the patient's issue to careful consideration of the treatment options. The model also includes a specific clinical application: the use of the mindful, experience-based cognitive process to determine whether an indwelling urinary catheter should be used. It seemed a particularly appropriate application since the important infection prevention strategy is essentially intellectual and behavioral rather than technical. Mindful clinicians will support the removal of indwelling urinary catheters as soon as possible because they know it will not only prevent urinary tract infections and reduce patients' discomfort, but also increase their mobility and independence, steps toward their leaving the hospital earlier. As well, mindful clinicians will think carefully about whether a central line is truly warranted, or if testing for C. difficile would change their management or have an impact on clinical care. Taking a moment to pause, reflect, assess

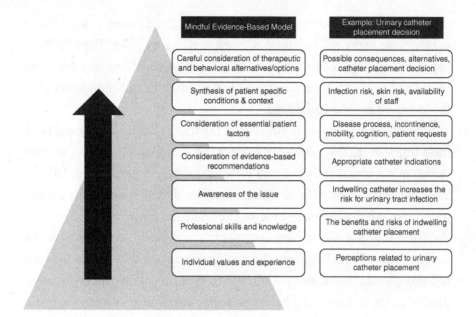

Mindful Evidence-Based Model	Example: Urinary catheter placement decision
Careful consideration of therapeutic and behavioral alternatives/options	Possible consequences, alternatives, catheter placement decision
Synthesis of patient specific conditions & context	Infection risk, skin risk, availability of staff
Consideration of essential patient factors	Disease process, incontinence, mobility, cognition, patient requests
Consideration of evidence-based recommendations	Appropriate catheter indications
Awareness of the issue	Indwelling catheter increases the risk for urinary tract infection
Professional skills and knowledge	The benefits and risks of indwelling catheter placement
Individual values and experience	Perceptions related to urinary catheter placement

Figure 11.1 Mindful evidence-based model. (From Kiyoshi-Teo et al.[42])

one's mental and emotional state, and think about thinking can have profound impact on behavior.

We conducted a study to explore the impact of a brief mindfulness training session on the hand hygiene behavior of four eight-person physician teams in a tertiary care health system. Two of the teams attended an hour-long session that included a video and a lecture by the chief investigator describing how he uses the principles of mindfulness to create moments of reflection while providing clinical care. These teams were provided with a document that had an overview of how mindfulness may be used while performing hand hygiene[43] to anchor the discussion within specific steps. The other two teams, controls, received no mindfulness instruction or document to support behavior change. Morning rounds on the medical wards were chosen as the testing venue.

Using a standardized, secret-shopper auditing approach, five observers developed baseline hand hygiene rates for the four teams both before and after their members interacted with patients. The observers were instructed that mindfulness behaviors could be identified in two ways: (1)

if the subject halted other activities to focus on handwashing or (2) if that person took many deliberate, slow breaths while washing. The observers kept tabs on all the teams for a period of five days, and team members also completed a mindfulness awareness test at baseline and then again after the intervention was completed.

In terms of hand hygiene adherence, the trial's results were by and large most impressive. The adherence rate for the attending physicians who received mindfulness training rose 14%, while their control group fell 6%. The interns in the mindfulness teams improved by 10%, while the control group increased adherence by 4%. The residents improved by 25%, and the control group saw no improvement. The medical students were the outliers—their hand hygiene adherence rate rose just 4.7%, while the control group's rate increased by 7.7%.[43] There were no significant changes indicated in the results of the before and after mindfulness awareness tests.

Focus groups and interviews were conducted with the two teams that received mindfulness training to explore their views on the intervention and on the experience of using mindfulness during hand hygiene. The teams were also asked for their recommendations for future implementations. Focus groups were used with the residents, interns, and medical students; the attendings were interviewed one on one. All of the participants expressed positive views concerning the use of mindfulness in clinical settings and its potential for improving physicians' sense of well-being and, thereby, their relationship with patients.

Some participants who liked the idea of practicing mindfulness during hand hygiene admitted that it was difficult because of the pressures of rounds. "Usually there were three other people behind me," an intern said, "and I thought it would be a little strange to just sit there pausing and thinking while everybody waited to go into the patient room." A resident suggested that attendings should take the lead in mindfulness practice: "If the attending stands outside the room and finishes washing his or her hands with the sanitizer, the rest of the team may actually pause there with him or her to do that."

On a personal level, in our role as mentors to many hundreds of doctors in training, we have found that mindfulness has greatly helped us cope with the inevitable challenges. Mentees often show up late for meetings. They overpromise and underdeliver. They indicate by their behavior that they would prefer another mentor. Mindfulness practice has enabled us to be patient, focused on the moment, and accepting of what happens with our mentees. It has been a boon to them—and to us!

THE POTENTIAL OF MOTIVATIONAL INTERVIEWING

How do you convince recalcitrant patients to give up smoking, start exercising, or watch their diet? Traditional forms of persuasion, in which you present all the logical reasons for behavior modification, may temporarily lead patients to new insights and a determination to change their ways, but the benefits of jawboning are typically brief. Too often, the bad habits triumph over the patients' good intentions.

Enter motivational interviewing (MI). It plays to patients' good intentions. The MI interviewer uses questions to identify patients' core values and helps them recognize how their current behavior fails to align with those values. Over the last decade, the use of MI as a counseling tool has won substantial acceptance in hospitals across the country.

But patients are not the only people in the hospital setting who may have trouble changing ill-advised behavior. We believe that MI could play an important role in winning over hospital staff members who resist evidence-based, quality improvement interventions. In fact, a pilot test using MI to improve hand hygiene among nurses at a university hospital in Iran has had promising preliminary results—though of course larger testing is needed.

An MI practitioner working with a patient starts by asking open-ended questions to find out how she feels about changing her behavior. The practitioner listens carefully to each answer and responds with a nonjudgmental rephrasing of the patient's observations and beliefs. The practitioner then asks the patient's permission to bring new information into the conversation, including aspects of the proposed change that have not been mentioned. The new information might be the mortality rate increases associated with

obesity or with smoking. The patient is led to recognize her own ambivalence about the matter—her reluctance to change versus her fears of an early
death and how that would affect her children. At the conclusion of a successful session, the patient begins to consider ways to adjust her life to the
changed behavior. And what is most important, the decision has not been
forced on her; she has made it herself, so it is more likely to stick.

We have developed two model MI exchanges to suggest how the technique might be applied with hospital staff who are resisting quality improvement initiatives: one on behalf of CAUTI prevention, the other to
improve hand hygiene.

Catheter-Associated Urinary Tract Infection

The scene: The office of the chief medical officer (CMO) of an acute care
hospital, late afternoon. A surgeon has entered the office and is now seated
across from the CMO.

> *Chief Medical Officer:* Thanks for coming over, Jim. I know you're
>   under the gun with all the staff cuts, but I do need to ask you
>   about something. I hear you've been having some trouble with
>   the new CAUTI initiative. Want to tell me about it?
>
> *Surgeon:* You bet I do. I've been ordering Foleys for 25 years, no
>   problem, and now they come along with all these new rules. It's
>   confusing. As far as I'm concerned, if it ain't broke, don't fix it.
>   And if I'm confused, just think about the poor residents who
>   have to unlearn what they've just been taught.
>
> *CMO:* I can see you're really frustrated about this. What else
>   bothers you about the new rules?
>
> *Surgeon:* You really want to know? How about this: I've got nurses
>   ordering me around! [Mimics female nurse] "Are you sure you
>   want to order that Foley, Doctor?" "Don't you think we should
>   remove that Foley now, Doctor?" Give me a break!

CMO: I get it, Jim. Tell me, what do you think about the science behind the initiative?

Surgeon: It sounds good, but you know they change their minds every few years. Meanwhile, we're supposed to dance to a new tune whenever another quality project shows up. Enough, already. And besides, why do I have to worry about urinary tract infections when I'm trying to save peoples' lives?

CMO: I hear you, loud and clear, and I appreciate how open you're being with me. One other thing, Jim. I wonder if you've been getting any flak from your colleagues about this.

Surgeon: Maybe a little. From some of the nurses, for sure, and I guess a few of the younger surgeons have made comments. The ones who are really annoyed with me are the people leading the initiative.

CMO: You seem to be saying you feel uncomfortable about that.

Surgeon: Well, they're smart, decent people, and they're obviously committed to making the changes.

CMO: Speaking of which, I just got some new info about the initiative. Interested?

Surgeon: I suppose so.

CMO: Did you know our CAUTI rate was up again last month? It's true CAUTI doesn't kill many people, but it sure makes them unhappy for a while. And when we use antibiotics on them, here comes *C. difficile*, which *does* kill people.

Surgeon: I didn't realize our infection rate was such a problem. I guess it *is* something to worry about.

CMO: That's where the initiative fits in. We have these new studies I want to show you. The hospitals in the studies had big reductions in the CAUTI rate, and they used the same evidence-based changes our initiative is pushing. So, there's a real chance to get something accomplished here.

Surgeon: Yeah, yeah. Got it. I suppose I'm going to have to give in sooner or later, and it might as well be sooner.

Hand Hygiene

The scene: A small conference room in an urban hospital system, early morning. A nurse manager and one of her nurses, paper coffee cups in hand, sit across from each other at the long table.

> *Nurse manager:* So, Margie, you must be wondering what this is all about. As you know, we've been doing an internal audit, and we've discovered that you don't seem to be following our hand hygiene procedures. I was hoping to hear how you feel about this.
>
> *Nurse:* It's not that I don't want to wash my hands, but the sanitizers are empty most of the time. Or they're way down the hall and the next patient is waiting for me.
>
> *Nurse manager:* It seems as though you understand how important handwashing is, but there are things that keep you from doing it. What else is there?
>
> *Nurse:* There are so many things. For example, we keep running out of supplies, which means I end up spending hours every day carrying them around, and it's hard to put them down to wash your hands. I keep bringing this up, but it doesn't change.
>
> *Nurse manager:* It sounds like you're frustrated because basic things aren't taken care of and that makes it hard for you to do your part.
>
> *Nurse:* Yeah, exactly.
>
> *Nurse manager:* Tell me what you remember from the hand hygiene training you've had.
>
> *Nurse:* Well, I know how the micro-organisms can move from our skin to a patient's skin and that sort of thing. And I know infection control is a priority. But we have so many priorities. Like all those questions we have to go over with a patient every single time we go into the room. There's just not enough time for everything. We're supposed to do more and more in the same amount of time.

Nurse manager: It sounds as if you understand the importance of infection control procedures, but time management problems keep you from following them.

Nurse: Yes. And sometimes those rules just don't make sense. Like if I'm delivering a blanket or a cup of water, it's not really patient care, so there's no need to wash my hands again.

Nurse manager: I can see that you are trying to be practical, given all the pressures on your time. Would it be OK with you if I shared some infection control data with you, and if we talked about ways to resolve some of your problems?

Nurse: Yeah, I guess, but it feels like I've been over this so many times.

Nurse manager: You're not sure more talk would accomplish anything?

Nurse: Yes, exactly. We have so many meetings and huddles around here, but nothing changes.

Nurse manager: Maybe you could help us find a better way to mobilize people around the hand hygiene program. For example, we need to find ways to present the infection control data so it's more meaningful to people. We need to find ways to make it easier for everyone to follow the hand hygiene protocols.

Nurse: I think if we could have our own workgroup, we would have some ideas, and if the leadership would actually support one of our ideas, it would be a big boost in our morale about everything, including hand hygiene.

Nurse manager: I appreciate your feedback, Margie. I know you understand that if we're not careful about hand hygiene, more of our patients will become infected. So, when our audit finds that the procedures are not being followed, we need to find out why.

Nurse: I do understand. For sure, I don't want something I did or didn't do to hurt my patients.

Though we believe that MI has the potential to help change behaviors in the clinical environment, we recognize that there are significant barriers to its large-scale deployment. Chief among them is the task of training substantial numbers of medical students in the practice of MI and validating such training by evaluating MI skills in the hospital setting. That said, the fact remains that many quality improvement initiatives fall short of their goals because of inadequate staff compliance—and it would be shortsighted to ignore any approach that could help correct that failing.

* * *

In this chapter, we have had the audacity to offer some thoughts about what the field of infection prevention might look like in the decades to come. As the great management guru Peter Drucker once commented, "Trying to predict the future is like trying to drive down a country road at night with no lights on while looking out the back window." We recognize that we have only lightly touched on the multitude of technical advances that are in development. On the adaptive side, in particular, what we have written here about the future represents our hopes at least as much as our expectations.

One item we have neglected to mention that does not represent our hopes, but that seems to be an inevitable part of the future of medicine, is IBM's Watson computer. IBM claims that the Watson can take in and analyze huge amounts of data better than humans, including physicians, and is thus just about ready to start making medical diagnoses. When confronted with a patient, the computer will be able to call up any and all of the relevant peer-reviewed medical knowledge of the past, as well as the latest research, all this to a degree no human doctor can match. This ability, one study found,[44] enabled Watson to achieve a 90% accuracy in diagnosing lung cancer, versus 50% for human physicians. By deriving the right diagnosis, the computer is touted as a means to drastically cut healthcare costs.

Presumably, within a decade or two, some combination of Watson and a robot will be deciding whether a central line or a urinary catheter should be placed or removed and will then fit the action to the word. What we find hard to imagine, though, is how this device will interact with patients. It doesn't seem to leave much room for patient empowerment, or for the human empathic and intuitive powers that machines—so far, at least— have been unable to muster.

In closing, we would like to thank you for joining us on this journey. If what you have read has helped you to move forward in your struggle to conquer HAI, our mission will have been achieved.

SUGGESTIONS FOR FURTHER READING

Borg MA. Cultural determinants of infection control behaviour: understanding drivers and implementing effective change. J Hosp Infect. 2014;86:161–168.

In this article, the author focused on three Hofstede constructs as necessary for improving infection prevention and control campaigns. In particular, he noted that many current infection prevention tools are strongly compatible with cultures that are low in uncertainty avoidance and power distance and high in individualism and masculinity, a cultural combination that is largely restricted to Anglo-Saxon countries, where most of the recent improvements in HAI incidence have taken place.

Cao J, Min L, Lansing B, Foxman B, Mody L. Multidrug-resistant organisms on patients' hands: a missed opportunity. JAMA Intern Med. 2016;176:705–706.

In this article, the authors revealed the increasing prevalence of multidrug-resistant organisms (MDROs) transmission in postacute care facilities through swab testing patient hands at monthly intervals. Due to the nature of postacute care facilities—where assistance may be needed for daily activities and mobility outside of room is encouraged—patients are at increased risk for MDRO cross transmission. Enforcement of routine patient handwashing is important for reducing these risks.

Kiyoshi-Teo H, Krein SL, Saint S. Applying mindful evidence-based practice at the bedside: using catheter-associated urinary tract infection as a model. Infect Control Hosp Epidemiol. 2013;34:1099–1101.

In this article, the authors introduced a mindful, evidence-based practice model that illustrates how mindfulness might be used to incorporate evidence-based practices into patient care at the individual clinician level. Using CAUTI prevention as an example, they illustrated how clinicians can be more mindful about appropriate catheter indications and timely catheter removal.

Patel PK, Mantey J, Mody L. Patient hand colonization with MDROs is associated with environmental contamination in post-acute care. Infect Control Hosp Epidemiol. 2017;38:1110–1113.

Patients with disability, urinary catheter, recent antibiotic use, and prolonged hospital stay are at risk for MDRO hand colonization. These risks are common for patients within postacute care facilities, and patient hand colonization was significantly associated with environmental contamination.

Petrilli CM, Mack M, Petrilli JJ, Hickner A, Saint S, Chopra V. Understanding the role of physician attire on patient perceptions: a systematic review of the literature—Targeting Attire to Improve Likelihood of Rapport (TAILOR) investigators. BMJ Open. 2015;5:e006578.

This systematic review of the literature examined the influence that physician attire has on patient perceptions, including trust, satisfaction, and confidence in providers. The review spanned 30 studies covering patients from 14 countries and found that while formal attire with a white coat is generally preferred, results may differ based on patient age, location, and care setting.

Petrilli CM, Saint S, Jennings JJ, et al. Understanding patient preference for physician attire: a cross-sectional observational study of 10 academic medical centres in the USA. BMJ Open. 2018;8:e021239.

The authors of this article sought out whether physician attire would affect patient experience and satisfaction. Based on 10 academic hospitals across the nation, 53% of patient responses indicated that physician attire was important, and one third agreed that it influenced their satisfaction with care. Perceptions of physician dress may vary depending on clinical context and region.

Saint S, Gaies E, Fowler KE, Harrod M, Krein SL. Introducing a catheter-associated urinary tract infection (CAUTI) prevention guide to patient safety (GPS). Am J Infect Control. 2014;42:548–550.

Based on extensive qualitative evaluations, the authors developed a self-assessment tool called a CAUTI Guide to Patient Safety (or "CAUTI GPS"). In this article, they described the rationale, features, and utility of such a quality improvement tool.

Saint S, Trautner BW, Fowler KE, et al. A multicenter study of patient-reported infectious and noninfectious complications associated with indwelling urethral catheters. JAMA Intern Med. 2018;178:1078–1085.

This study, including over 2,000 patients across four US hospitals, followed up with patients 30 days after urinary catheter insertion to determine the incidence of infectious and noninfectious harms associated with the use of an indwelling catheter. Fifty-seven percent reported at least one complication. Of those, 55% reported noninfectious complications, such as pain or discomfort, blood in the urine, and the like. These lesser known complications underscore the need for prompt urinary catheter removal.

Salmon P, Hall GM. Patient empowerment or the emperor's new clothes. J R Soc Med. 2004;97:53–56.

In this article, Salmon and Hall explored the validity of "empowerment" as a concept by studying the experience of patients who have been empowered to take control and make choices. Based on these accounts from the patients' perspective, the authors suggested that patients do not generally embrace empowerment, and that, in emphasizing research into how to empower patients at the expense of research into what patients feel like when they have been empowered, medicine paradoxically continues the tradition of assuming that doctor knows best.

Spellberg B, Bartlett JG, Gilbert DN. The future of antibiotics and resistance. N Engl J Med. 2013;368:299–302.

In this article, the authors proposed future strategies to combat antimicrobial resistance. They suggested that long-term solutions require novel approaches based on a reconceptualization of the nature of resistance, disease, and prevention, and that additional societal investment in basic and applied research and policy activities is imperative.

Ann Arbor Criteria for Urinary Catheters
in Hospitalized Medical Patients

Box A.1

GUIDE FOR FOLEY CATHETER USE IN HOSPITALIZED MEDICAL PATIENTS*

A. Appropriate Indications for Foley Catheter Use
Acute urinary retention without bladder outlet obstruction.
  Example: medication-related urinary retention

Acute urinary retention with bladder outlet obstruction due to non-infectious, non-traumatic diagnosis
  Example: exacerbation of benign prostatic hyperplasia
  Caution: consider urology consultation for catheter type and/or placement for conditions such as acute prostatitis and urethral trauma

Chronic urinary retention with bladder outlet obstruction**

Stage III, IV or unstageable pressure ulcers or similarly severe wounds of other types that cannot be kept clear of urinary incontinence despite wound care and other urinary management strategies[a]

Urinary incontinence in patients with substantial difficulty by nurses to provide skin care despite other urinary management strategies[a] and available resources such as lift teams and mechanical lift devices
  Examples: turning causes hemodynamic or respiratory instability, strict prolonged immobility (such as in unstable spine or pelvic fractures), strict temporary immobility post-procedure (such as after vascular

catheterization), or excess weight (>300 pounds) from severe edema or obesity

Hourly measurement of urine volume is required to provide treatment

Examples: manage hemodynamic instability, hourly titration of fluids, drips (e.g., vasopressors, inotropes) or life-supportive therapy

Daily (not hourly) measurement of urine volume is required to provide treatment and cannot be assessed by other volume[b] and urine collection strategies[c]

Examples: acute renal failure work-up, IVF or acute IV or oral diuretic management, fluid management in respiratory failure

Single 24-hour urine sample for diagnostic test when cannot be obtained by other urine collection strategies[c]

Reduce <u>acute</u>, severe pain with movement when difficulty with other urine management strategies[a]

Example: acute unrepaired fracture

Improve comfort when urine collection by catheter addresses patient and family goals in a dying patient

Management of gross hematuria with blood clots in urine

Clinical condition for which ISC or external condom catheter would be appropriate however placement was difficult by experienced nurse or physician and/or had inadequate bladder emptying with non-indwelling strategies during this admission

B. Inappropriate Uses of Foley Catheters

Urinary incontinence when nurses can turn/provide skin care with available resources, including patients with intact skin, incontinence-associated dermatitis, and pressure ulcers stages I, II and closed deep tissue injury.

Routine use of Foley in ICU without an appropriate indication

Foley placement to reduce risk of falls by minimizing the need to get up to urinate

Post-void residual urine volume assessment

Random or 24 urine sample collection for sterile or non-sterile specimens if possible by other collection strategies[c]

Patient[***] or family request when no expected difficulties managing urine otherwise in non-dying patient, including during patient transport

Patient is ordered for "bed rest" without strict immobility requirement

    Example: lower extremity cellulitis or injury

To prevent urinary tract infection (UTI) in patient with fecal incontinence or diarrhea, or to manage frequent, painful urination in patients with UTI

Reprinted with permission from *Annals of Internal Medicine*.[1]

[*] This table provides guidance for Foley catheter use in the medical patient, excluding both appropriate and inappropriate uses in the peri-operative setting.

[**] It is unclear if a Foley catheter is appropriate for chronic urinary retention without bladder outlet obstruction (e.g., neurogenic bladder) when ISC is feasible and adequate; appropriateness may vary based on reason for urinary retention, and level of difficulty or discomfort performing ISC.

[***] It is unclear if a Foley is appropriate for a patient who chronically uses ISC but requests "break" from ISC by using Foley while admitted because transition to Foley may lead to difficulties returning to ISC regimen as outpatient, but it is acknowledged that a patient's clinical capabilities to perform self-catheterization may be reduced based upon reason for admission, and patient with self-catheterization history may prefer to avoid catheterization by others.

[a] Other urinary <u>management</u> strategies: barrier creams, absorbent pads, prompted toileting, non-indwelling catheters

[b] Other <u>volume assessment</u> strategies: physical exam, daily weights

[c] Other urine <u>collection</u> strategies: urinal, bedside commode, bedpan, external catheter

Abbreviations: ISC, intermittent straight catheter; IVF, intravenous fluid; IV, intravenous

Box A.2

GUIDE FOR INTERMITTENT STRAIGHT CATHETERIZATION (ISC) IN HOSPITALIZED MEDICAL PATIENTS

A. Appropriate Indications for ISC*

Acute urinary retention without bladder outlet obstruction, if bladder can be emptied adequately by at maximum frequency of ISC every 4 hours

> *Example: medication-related urinary retention*

Acute urinary retention with bladder outlet obstruction due to non-infectious, non-traumatic diagnosis.

> *Example: exacerbation of benign prostatic hyperplasia*
> *Caution: consider urology consultation for catheter type and/or placement for conditions such as acute prostatitis or urethral trauma*

Chronic urinary retention with or without bladder outlet obstruction

Stage III, IV or unstageable pressure ulcers or similarly severe wounds of other types that cannot be kept clear of urinary incontinence despite wound care and other urinary management strategies[a] if ISC is adequate to manage the type of incontinence (i.e., overflow)

Urinary incontinence that is treated and can be managed by ISC (i.e., overflow incontinence)

Urine volume measurements (not hourly) or sample collections in patients using ISC for urinary retention/obstruction or overflow incontinence

Random urine sample collection for sterile or non-sterile specimens if impossible by other collection strategies[b]

To manage urine in patients with strict temporary immobility if performing ISC does not require excessive movement

Post-void residual urine volume assessment if bladder scanner is unavailable or inadequate, and more detail is needed than suprapubic fullness

B. Inappropriate Uses of ISC

Hourly measurement of urine volume is required to provide treatment

Random urine sample collection for sterile or non-sterile samples if possible by other strategies[c]

Reprinted with permission from *Annals of Internal Medicine*.[1]

* It is unclear if ISC is an appropriate option to try for urinary management in distressed patients such as those with dyspnea or end-of-life due to concerns that potential discomfort from ISC could add to distress.

[a] Other urinary <u>management</u> strategies: barrier creams, absorbent pads, prompted toileting, external catheters

[b] Other urine <u>collection</u> strategies: urinal, bedside commode, bedpan, external catheter

---

Box A.3

GUIDE FOR EXTERNAL CATHETER USE* IN HOSPITALIZED MEDICAL PATIENTS

A. Appropriate Indications for External Catheters

Stage III, IV or unstageable pressure ulcers or similarly severe wounds of other types that cannot be kept clear of urinary incontinence despite wound care and other urinary management strategies[a] **

Moderate-severe incontinence-associated dermatitis that cannot be kept clear of urine despite other urinary management strategies[a]

Urinary incontinence in patients with substantial difficulty by nurses to provide skin care despite other urinary management strategies[a] and available resources such as lift teams and mechanical lift devices

> *Examples: turning causes hemodynamic or respiratory instability, strict prolonged immobility (such as in unstable spine or pelvic fractures), strict temporary immobility post-procedure (such as after vascular catheterization), or excess weight (>300 pounds) from severe edema or obesity*

Daily (not hourly) measurement of urine volume is required to provide treatment and cannot be assessed by other volume[b] and urine collection strategies[c]

> *Examples: acute renal failure work-up, IVF or acute IV or oral diuretic management, fluid management in respiratory failure*

Single 24-hour or random sterile*** or non-sterile urine sample for diagnostic test when cannot be obtained by other urine collection strategies[c]

Reduce <u>acute</u>, severe pain with movement when difficulty with other urine management strategies[a]

> *Example: acute unrepaired fracture*

Patient request for external catheter to manage urinary incontinence while hospitalized

Improve comfort when urine collection by catheter addresses patient and family goals in a dying patient

B. Inappropriate Uses for External Catheters

Any use in a non-cooperative patient expected to frequently manipulate catheters due to behavior issues like delirium, dementia

Any type of urinary retention (acute or chronic, with or without bladder outlet obstruction)

Hourly measurement of urine volume is required to provide treatment

Urinary incontinence when nurses can turn/provide skin care with available resources, including patients with intact skin, incontinence-associated dermatitis, and pressure ulcers stages I, II and closed deep tissue injury

Routine use in ICU without an appropriate indication

External catheter placement to reduce risk of falls by minimizing the need to get up to urinate

Post-void residual urine volume assessment

24-hour or random sample collection for sterile*** or non-sterile specimens if possible by non-catheter collection strategies[c]

Foley placement for convenience of urinary management in patient during transport for tests and procedures

Patient or family request when no expected difficulties managing urine in non-dying patient

To prevent urinary tract infection (UTI) in patient with fecal incontinence or diarrhea, or to manage frequent, painful urination in patients with UTI

Reprinted with permission from *Annals of Internal Medicine*.[1]

* Note: At time of this publication, external catheters are primarily developed and used for male patients in the form of condom catheters. However, these indications would also be applicable to female patients after development of external catheters appropriate and adequate for female patients.

** It is unclear if external catheters are appropriate for early/mild incontinence associated dermatitis or incontinence with early stage pressure ulcers (stage I, II, closed deep tissue injury), due to the increased risk of infection even with external catheters, and availability of non-catheter strategies to manage urinary incontinence, balanced.

***Sterile sample collection using external catheter is feasible and appropriate but ability to perform is dependent upon clinician experience

[a] Other urinary management strategies: barrier creams, absorbent pads, prompted toileting

[b] Other volume assessment strategies: physical exam, daily weights

[c] Other urine collection strategies: urinal, bedside commode, bedpan

Table A.1 SUMMARY FOR MOST COMMON USES OF FOLEY, ISC, AND EXTERNAL CATHETERS

Is this reason an appropriate clinical indication for catheter use?	Foley indwelling urinary catheter	Intermittent straight catheter (ISC)	External condom catheter	Non-catheter options
1. PATIENT CANNOT URINATE DUE TO URINARY RETENTION				
Acute retention WITHOUT bladder outlet obstruction *Examples: medication related (opioids, anticholinergics, paralytics)*	Yes	Yes, if bladder can be emptied by 4–6 hour ISC	No, cannot address urinary retention	Bladder scanner, to avoid catheterizing when no or little urine seen in bladder
Acute retention WITH bladder outlet obstruction	Foley/ISC appropriateness vary by obstruction type *Consider Urology consultation for prostatitis, urethral trauma.*			
Chronic urinary retention WITHOUT bladder outlet obstruction	Uncertain+	Yes		
Chronic urinary retention WITH bladder outlet obstruction	Yes	Yes		
2. PATIENT CANNOT STOP OR CONTROL URINATION *due to incontinence*				
Incontinence (no skin issue), nurses can turn/provide skin care	No	No	No	Barrier creams, prompted toileting, garments can often manage incontinence-related skin issues.
Incontinence, can be turned, patient requests catheter	No	No	Uncertain+	
Incontinence (no skin issues), difficulty turning due to: *Excess weight (>300 pounds) from obesity or edema*	Yes	No	Yes	

Turning causes hemodynamic or respiratory instability	Yes	No	Yes	
Strict temporary immobility after vascular procedure	Yes. All catheters appropriate if cannot manage urine otherwise.			
Incontinence with mild/early incontinence-associated dermatitis	No	No	Uncertain+	
Incontinence with mod/severe incontinence-associated dermatitis	No	No	Yes	
Incontinence with closed pressure ulcer: stage I, deep tissue injury	No	No	Uncertain+	Yes, if would not worsen ulcer
Incontinence with open pressure ulcer stage II	No	Yes if ISC is adequate to manage the incontinence	Uncertain+	
Incontinence with open pressure ulcer stage III, IV, or unstageable	Yes	Yes	Yes	
*3. CLINICIAN REQUESTS CATHETER TO MEASURE URINE VOLUME**				
Hourly urine volume is required to provide treatment. *Example: manage hemodynamic instability; hourly titrate IVF, drips*	Yes	No	No	No
Daily (not hourly) urine volume required to guide treatment. *Examples: acute renal failure work-up, IVF or oral/IV bolus diuretics, fluid management in respiratory failure*	Yes, if cannot be collected/assessed without catheter	Uncertain+	Yes, if cannot assess without catheter	Exam/daily weight. Urinal, bedpan, etc.

Table A.1 CONTINUED

Is this reason an appropriate clinical indication for catheter use?	Foley indwelling urinary catheter	Intermittent straight catheter (ISC)	External condom catheter	Non-catheter options
Post-void residual urine volume	No	Yes, if no bladder scanner	No	Bladder scanner
4. URINE SPECIMEN COLLECTION IS NEEDED TO PERFORM A DIAGNOSTIC TEST**				
Sterile sample for urine culture	No	Yes	Uncertain+	No
Non-sterile random urine sample	No	Yes	Yes	No
24-hour urine sample	Yes	Uncertain++	Yes	No
5. URINE CATHETER IS REQUESTED TO PROVIDE COMFORT AND/OR CONVENIENCE				
Improve comfort (address patient/family goals) in dying patient	Yes	Uncertain++	Yes	Yes, for all options
Family or patient request in non-dying patient with no incontinence or difficulties using commode, urinal or bedpan	No	No	No	Yes, for all options
Chronic ISC patient requests a "break" from ISC while admitted	Uncertain++	Yes	No	Bladder scanner

Reprinted with permission from *Annals of Internal Medicine*.[1]

* It is *inappropriate* to use a urinary catheter simply because the patient is being cared for in an intensive care unit; an appropriate medical indication is required

** When *cannot* be collected by non-catheter means;

+ Uncertain due to disagreement between panelist ratings

++ Uncertain due to panelist ratings having median score of 4–6

Is the Foley catheter still appropriate for your ICU patient? If your patient does not have one of the following criteria, remove Foley catheter.

1. Urine volume measurement:

    a. Is HOURLY urine volume measurement being used to inform and provide treatment? Examples:

      Hemodynamic instability requiring hourly or multiple daily titrations per day of ongoing bolus fluid resuscitation, vasopressors, inotropes, or diuretics

      Acute respiratory failure requiring invasive ventilation with hourly titrations of diuretics

      Hourly measurement of urine studies or urine volumes to manage life-threatening laboratory abnormalities

    b. Is DAILY urine volume measurement being used to provide treatment AND volume status CANNOT be adequately or reliably assessed without a Foley catheter, such as by daily weight or urine collection by urinal, commode, bedpan, or external catheter? Examples:

      Management of acute renal failure, IV fluids, or IV or oral bolus diuretics

      Fluid management in acute respiratory failure requiring large volumes of oxygen (≥5 L/min or >50%)

2. Does patient have a urologic problem that is being treated with a Foley catheter? Examples:

      Urinary retention that cannot be adequately monitored or addressed by bladder scanner or ISC

      Urinary retention anticipated because of treatment with paralytic medications

      Recent urologic or gynecologic evaluation or procedure with Foley catheter not recommended to be removed yet, such as:
      - Acute urinary retention with bladder outlet obstruction due to acute prostatitis or urethral edema
      - Gross hematuria with blood clots in the urine
      - Hematuria suspected to be prostatic or urethral bleeding being managed with Foley catheter

3. Urine sample collection for a laboratory test when CANNOT be collected by non-catheter method

What type of sample is needed?	Use Foley Catheter?	Use ISC?	Use External Catheter?
Sterile sample for urine culture	No	Yes	Yes, if staff trained for sterile application
Non-sterile random urine sample	No	Yes	Yes
24-hour urine sample	Yes	If all urine can be collected by ISC	Yes, preferred option in cooperative males External female catheters also able to collect and measure 24-hour urine volumes; there is no published literature yet regarding the impact of the external female catheter materials on the results of the urine tests.

4. Does the patient have urinary incontinence that cannot be addressed by non-catheter methods (barrier creams, incontinence garments and absorbent pads, prompted toileting, straight catheterization if overflow incontinence) because nurses cannot turn and provide skin care with specialty resources (such as lift teams and lift machines) or transition to external catheter (for cooperative males)? Examples:

      Turning causes hemodynamic or respiratory instability

      Strict temporary immobility post procedure, such as from a vascular procedure if patient cannot manage urine otherwise

      Incontinence with open pressure ulcers (stage III or IV) or "unstageable" ulcers

5. Foley catheter is providing comfort from severe distress related to urinary management that cannot be addressed by non-catheter options, ISC, or external catheter. Examples:

      Difficulty voiding due to severe dyspnea with position changes required for managing urine without an indwelling catheter

      Address patient and family goals in a dying patient

      Acute, severe pain upon movement (e.g., unrepaired fracture) WITH demonstrated difficulties using non-catheter options or external catheter

ICU=intensive care unit; ISC=intermittent straight catheter; IV=intravenous.

Figure A.1 Intensive care unit daily checklist for appropriateness of Foley catheter. (Reprinted with permission from *Annals of Internal Medicine*.[1])

APPENDIX B

Michigan Appropriate Perioperative (MAP) Criteria for Urinary Catheter Use

Table B.1 SUMMARY OF PERIOPERATIVE URINARY CATHETER USE RECOMMENDATIONS[A]

A. *Avoid placing indwelling urinary catheters for these routine procedures:* these are procedures for which it is considered inappropriate to place a catheter for the procedure, as the catheter risk is considered to outweigh the benefits for the patient.[b, c]

General Surgery	Orthopedic Surgery
• Laparoscopic cholecystectomy	• Unilateral total knee arthroplasty
• Open appendectomy	• Unilateral/bilateral unicompartmental knee arthroplasty
• Laparoscopic appendectomy without suprapubic port	• Unilateral osteotomy for unicompartmental or non-inflammatory knee disease
• Open reducible inguinal, femoral, umbilical or epigastric hernia repair	• Revision knee arthroplasty, to last ≤ 2 hours
• Laparoscopic reducible inguinal or femoral hernia repair by TAPP if bladder emptied before surgery	• Unilateral (not revision) total prosthetic hip replacement (total hip arthroplasty)
• Laparoscopic reducible umbilical or epigastric hernia repair	• Unilateral closed reduction percutaneous pinning for femoral neck fracture
• Laparoscopic adjustable gastric banding	

(continued)

B. *Procedures to consider removing indwelling urinary catheter before leaving the OR*	
General Surgery • Laparoscopic reducible inguinal or femoral hernia by TEP approach • Laparoscopic Roux-en-Y gastric bypass[d] • Laparoscopic sleeve gastrectomy[d] • Open or laparoscopic ileocecectomy, hemicolectomy (right, transverse or left), or sigmoidectomy[d] • Laparoscopic subtotal colectomy[d]	Orthopedic Surgery • Bilateral total knee arthroplasty[d] • Revision knee arthroplasty, to last > 2 hours[d] • Unilateral partial prosthetic hip replacement[d] • Unilateral open reduction and internal fixation for hip fracture[d] • Unilateral total prosthetic replacement for hip fracture[d] • Bilateral total hip replacement/arthroplasty[d] • Revision prosthetic hip replacement[d]
C. *Procedures in which urinary catheter use in the OR and until at least postoperative day 1 is appropriate, with the timing for first trial of void detailed below by procedure*	
General Surgery • Laparoscopic biliopancreatic diversion with duodenal switch (postoperative day 1)[e] • Open subtotal colectomy (postoperative day 1) • Open or laparoscopic rectal resection of upper one-third of rectum[d] (post-op day 1) • Laparoscopic low anterior resection (postoperative day 1)[f] • Open abdominal perineal resection (postoperative day 2)[g] • Open or laparoscopic total proctocolectomy[h]	Orthopedic Surgery • See Section B for procedures[d] in which removal on postoperative day 1 is also appropriate. It is inappropriate to wait until postoperative day 2 or later to remove catheters after routine hip or knee arthroplasty procedures, including hip fracture repair.

Reprinted with permission from BMJ Quality & Safety.[1]

Abbreviations: OR, operating room; TAPP, transabdominal preperitoneal; TEP, totally extraperitoneal

[a] These are recommendations for perioperative urinary catheter use for patients without another indication for urinary catheter use (e.g., not needed to address a medical indication such as critical illness for which hourly urine output is being used to guide therapy such as vasopressors). For all procedures, using a post-operative protocol to monitor and address urinary retention symptoms is recommended; bladder scanners are increasingly common tools to verify retention in patients with symptoms to avoid unnecessary catheterizations.

[b] Routine urinary catheter use is not appropriate for these procedures when less than 2 hours of OR time and less than 2 L of intravenous fluids anticipated in the OR. Experts indicated that routine catheter use during the OR case could be appropriate for procedures > 3 hours in duration or with > 3 liters of intraoperative fluids.

[c] Patients are recommended to void before surgery. If concerned about postvoid residual, use of bladder scanner protocol with intermittent straight catheter as needed before surgery is an appropriate alternative to routine indwelling catheter use in patients with urinary retention.

[d] For these procedures, it was assessed also as clinically appropriate to remove catheter on postoperative day 1.

[e] For this procedure, there was uncertainty about appropriateness of routinely removing on the same day of surgery; therefore, it could be clinically appropriate to remove earlier than postoperative day 1 by surgeon's discretion.

[f] For open low anterior resection, removal before postoperative day 3 is appropriate, but there was uncertainty for whether removal was more appropriate on postoperative day 1 compared to postoperative day 2.

[g] For laparoscopic abdominal perineal resection, removal by postoperative day 4 is appropriate, but there was uncertainty for whether a particular day within the range of postoperative days 1–4 was more appropriate than others.

[h] For open or laparoscopic total proctocolectomy with or without ileal pouch anal anastamosis, removal by postoperative day 4 is appropriate, but there was uncertainty for whether a particular day within the range of postoperative days 1–4 was more appropriate than others.

Two-Tier Approach to Prioritize Interventions for
Catheter-Associated Urinary Tract Infection (CAUTI),
Central Line–Associated Bloodstream Infection (CLABSI),
and *Clostridioides difficile* Infection (CDI)

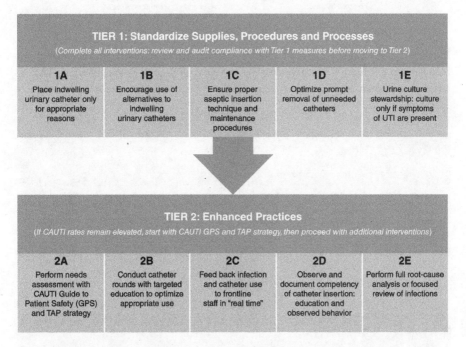

Figure C.1 Tiers of interventions to prevent CAUTI. CAUTI, catheter-associated urinary tract infection; GPS, guide to patient safety; TAP, targeted assessment for prevention; UTI, urinary tract infection. (Reprinted with permission from *Annals of Internal Medicine*.[1-3])

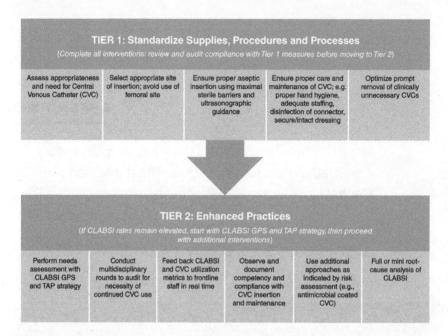

Figure C.2 Tiers of interventions to prevent CLABSI. CLABSI, central line-associated bloodstream infection; CVC, central venous catheter; GPS, guide to patient safety; TAP, targeted assessment for prevention. (Reprinted with permission from *Annals of Internal Medicine*.[2-4])

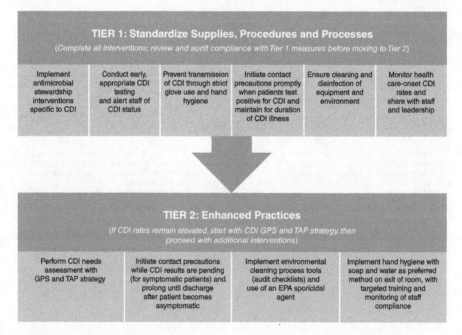

Figure C.3 Tiers of interventions to prevent CDI. CDI, *Clostridioides difficile* infection; GPS, guide to patient safety; TAP, targeted assessment for prevention. (Reprinted with permission from *Annals of Internal Medicine*.[2,3,5])

Guide to Patient Safety (GPS) Tools for CAUTI, CLABSI, and CDI

To accurately assess the organization's catheter-associated urinary tract infection (CAUTI) prevention efforts, it is recommended that:

1. The individual or team working on CAUTI prevention at the hospital or unit level completes the CAUTI GPS assessment. This can be done independently or as a group.
2. The responses are reviewed as a team if possible as a means to uncover strengths and barriers to reducing CAUTI.
3. For each question, if a response is chosen that reveals a barrier to reducing CAUTI, the text below gives guidance to review the approaches, advice, tools, or resources to better implement the CAUTI prevention strategy queried in that question.

Box D.1

CAUTI Guide to Patient Safety

1. Do you currently collect data related to CAUTI process measures (e.g., urinary catheter prevalence, urinary catheter appropriateness) or outcomes (e.g., CLABSI rates) in the unit(s) in which you are intervening?

☐ Yes   ☐ No

If you answered No, this implies that you do not currently collect data related to CAUTI prevention, such as days of catheter use or rates of infection. Collecting both pre- and postintervention data provides an objective way to evaluate if your interventions are successful in reducing CAUTI. Ongoing assessments allow you to evaluate if the intervention is sustained.

For additional tools, resources, and further reading, please visit our Preventing Hospital Infection Resource page at **https://psep.med.umich.edu/phi.html**

See section on Data Collection.

2. Do you routinely report CAUTI-related metrics and data to front-line staff and physicians (e.g., urinary catheter prevalence, urinary catheter appropriateness, and infection rates)?

☐ Yes   ☐ No

If you answered No, this implies that you do not routinely report CAUTI-related data to front-line staff. Staff awareness of CAUTI-related data is an important part of quality improvement. Hospitals have often found that transparency of sharing as much information as possible with staff can help staff stay motivated and engaged throughout the quality improvement initiative.

For additional tools, resources, and further reading, please visit our Preventing Hospital Infection Resource page at **https://psep.med.umich.edu/phi.html**

See section on Infection Prevention Feedback.

3. Do bedside nurses daily assess whether their catheterized patients still need a urinary catheter?

☐ Yes   ☐ No

If you answered No, this implies that bedside nurses either do not take the initiative or do not contact physicians to ensure that urinary catheters are removed when no longer clinically necessary. Necessity of an indwelling urinary catheter may change while a patient is in the hospital; therefore, it is imperative to continually assess its appropriateness.

For additional tools, resources, and further reading, please visit our Preventing Hospital Infection Resource page at **https://psep.med.umich.edu/phi.html**

See section on Catheter Necessity and Removal.

4. Do bedside nurses daily assess whether their catheterized patients still need a urinary catheter? If yes, do bedside nurses take initiative to remove the catheter when assessing as unnecessary (if empowered to do so) or have a systematic process to contact physicians to request an order to ensure the indwelling urinary catheter is removed when the catheter is no longer needed?

☐ Yes   ☐ No

If you answered No, this implies that bedside nurses either do not currently perform daily assessment of indwelling urinary catheter necessity or do not take the initiative to either remove it themselves when not necessary (if empowered) or contact physicians to ensure that urinary catheters are removed when no longer clinically necessary. Necessity of an indwelling urinary catheter may change while a patient is in the hospital; therefore, it is imperative to continually assess its appropriateness. Daily assessment of catheter necessity by the bedside nurse is one of the most important tools for reducing unnecessary catheter use, particularly because physicians may be unaware the catheter remains in place. Timely removal of the indwelling urinary catheter is crucial for reducing CAUTI; therefore, nurses should be empowered and supported to take the initiative of removing the catheter when it is no longer appropriate (e.g., by contacting the physician or removing the catheter per approved protocol).

For additional tools, resources, and further reading, please see **https://psep.med.umich.edu/phi.html**

See section on Catheter Necessity and Removal.

5. At your facility, are indwelling urinary catheters placed in response to requests by patients or family?

☐ Yes   ☐ No

If you answered Yes, this implies that patients and families often request urinary catheters in your facility. Educating patients and their family members about urinary catheter risks is important and may reduce unnecessary use. It is important to realize that patients and family may be requesting for convenience rather than an appropriate medical indication where the benefit outweighs the risks, and patients and family may not understand the short-term and long-term risks of urinary catheterization, including CAUTI, including potential serious multidrug-resistant infections or bacteremia, as well as the risks of urinary tract trauma from placement or removal (which may be as common or more common than infection), and the risks associated with reduced mobility when the patient is connected to an indwelling urinary catheter that serves as a "one-point restraint."

For additional tools, resources, and further reading, please visit our Preventing Hospital Infection Resource page at **https://psep.med.umich. edu/phi.html**

See section on Patient Education.

6. Have you experienced indwelling urinary catheters commonly being inserted in the emergency department without an appropriate indication?

☐ Yes   ☐ No

If you answered Yes, this implies that urinary catheters are inserted without an appropriate indication in your facility. In the unpredictable environment of the emergency department, nurses and doctors are more concerned about other patient concerns than about whether they have a catheter. It takes a member of the CAUTI prevention team to convince the emergency department that catheters count.

For additional tools, resources, and further reading, please visit our Preventing Hospital Infection Resource page at **https://psep.med.umich. edu/phi.html**

See section on Appropriateness.

7. Is the use of indwelling urinary catheters in your hospital restricted to a list of clinically appropriate indications?

☐ Yes   ☐ No

If you answered No, this implies that indwelling urinary catheter insertion is not restricted to clinically appropriate indications, meaning that patients may be receiving urinary catheters for reasons for which the risk of catheter-associated harm is likely to exceed the clinical benefits, such as for the convenience of the patient or the healthcare staff. In recent years, formal assessment of appropriateness for use of three types of urinary catheters (indwelling, external, and straight catheters) has been published to guide clinical use for hospitalized adults on medical services, as well as criteria for appropriate perioperative urinary catheter use for common general surgery and orthopedic surgery procedures. Prior studies have supported that catheters that are placed without an appropriate clinical indication are more likely to remain in place for prolonged periods, further increasing the risk of catheter-associated complications.

For additional tools, resources, and further reading, please visit our Preventing Hospital Infection Resource page at **https://psep.med.umich. edu/phi.html**

See section on Urinary Catheter Appropriateness Criteria.

8. Are external urinary catheters routinely used as alternatives to indwelling urinary catheters for men and women at your hospital?

☐ Yes   ☐ No

If you answered No, this implies that patients may be receiving indwelling catheters (and their higher associated risks of infectious and noninfections complications) when a safer alternative such as an external urinary catheter exists. External catheters have been available and routinely used for adult men in many hospitals (particular Veterans Administration hospitals in the United States) for many years, initially designed as condom-style catheters to collect urine but now with several other designs that may work better for certain patients. In recent years, there are also new external urinary catheter options for adult women that work well for managing urinary incontinence in women while in bed; the peer-reviewed literature describing the use and patient outcomes for external female urinary catheters is more limited but promising. External urinary catheters are good options to consider when additional help is needed to manage urinary incontinence or collect urine samples when other incontinence strategies (e.g., timed voiding, incontinence garments) are inadequate.

It is important to note external catheters can only collect spontaneously voided urine; they are inappropriate to use for a patient with urinary retention.

For additional tools, resources, and further reading, please visit our Preventing Hospital Infection Resource page at **https://psep.med.umich.edu/phi.html**

See section on Alternatives to Indwelling Urinary Catheters.

9. Do you have a well-functioning team focusing on CAUTI prevention?

☐ Yes   ☐ No

If you answered No, this implies either that you do not have a team or the one you have does not function well for preventing CAUTI. Because your CAUTI prevention team is responsible for defining, designing, leading, and sustaining the initiative, it is crucial that it functions well.

For additional tools, resources, and further reading, please visit our Preventing Hospital Infection Resource page at **https://psep.med.umich.edu/phi.html**

See section on Identifying a Team.

10. Do you have a team leader with dedicated time to coordinate CAUTI prevention activities?

☐ Yes   ☐ No

If you selected No, this indicates either that you do not have a team leader or that the one you have does not have appropriate time for CAUTI prevention. The team leader is responsible for many tasks, including coordinating and facilitating team meetings, communication, and overseeing team members. It is imperative that she or he has dedicated time to commit to the project.

For additional tools, resources, and further reading, please see **https://psep.med.umich.edu/phi.html**

See section on Identifying a Team Leader.

11. Do you have an effective nurse champion for CAUTI prevention activities?

☐ Yes   ☐ No

If you answered No, this implies either that you do not have a nurse champion or that the one you have is not effective when it comes to CAUTI prevention activities. A CAUTI initiative is dependent on nurses; therefore, getting their buy-in—with the help of an effective nurse champion—is key. The ideal nurse champion is well respected, trusted by peers, supportive of safety, and an agent of change.

For additional tools, resources, and further reading, please visit our Preventing Hospital Infection Resource page at **https://psep.med.umich. edu/phi.html**

See section on Identifying a Nurse Champion.

12. Do you have an effective physician champion for CAUTI prevention activities?

☐ Yes   ☐ No

If you answered No, this implies either that you do not have a physician champion for your CAUTI prevention activities or that the one you have is not effective. CAUTI prevention efforts require collaboration and support of both physicians and nurses, and an effective physician champion can lead change and win over physician colleagues.

For additional tools, resources, and further reading, please visit our Preventing Hospital Infection Resource page at **https://psep.med.umich. edu/phi.html**

See section on Identifying a Physician Champion.

13. Does senior leadership support your CAUTI prevention activities?

☐ Yes   ☐ No

If you answered No, this implies that you do not have the support of senior leadership for your CAUTI prevention activities. Prevention initiatives are costly and often require approval from managerial staff in departments such as medical executive leadership, purchasing, and accounts. It is helpful if hospital administrators and clinical chiefs take on personal leadership roles in quality improvement initiatives. Ideally, one member of the executive leadership team will be primarily responsible for overseeing the

CAUTI initiative at your hospital. In our experience, this often is the chief nursing executive.

For additional tools, resources, and further reading, please visit our Preventing Hospital Infection Resource page at **https://psep.med.umich. edu/phi.html**

See section on Senior Leadership Support.

14. Have you experienced substantial nursing resistance?

☐ Yes   ☐ No

If you answered Yes, this implies that you have experienced a lack of engagement or resistance from nursing staff. In a CAUTI prevention program, nursing and front-line staff are central to the success of the initiative. These staff are whose day-to-day activities are most affected by the changes, and therefore they may present the greatest resistance.

For additional tools, resources, and further reading, please visit our Preventing Hospital Infection Resource page at **https://psep.med.umich. edu/phi.html**

See section on Nurse Engagement.

15. Have you experienced substantial physician resistance?

☐ Yes   ☐ No

If you answered Yes, this implies that you have experienced a lack of engagement or resistance from physician staff. The daily operations of a quality improvement project require the ability of staff to adopt new goals and practices, and it is important that the physicians embrace and not resist the implementation of CAUTI prevention activities at your site/unit.

For additional tools, resources, and further reading, please visit our Preventing Hospital Infection Resource page at **https://psep.med.umich. edu/phi.html**

See section on Physician Engagement.

Source: Updated from Saint et al.[1-4]

To accurately assess the organization's central line–associated blood-stream infection (CLABSI) prevention efforts, it is recommended that:

1. The individual or team working on CLABSI prevention at the hospital or unit level complete the CLABSI GPS assessment. This can be done independently or as a group.
2. The responses are reviewed as a team as a means to uncover strengths and barriers to reducing CLABSI.
3. For each question, if a response is chosen that reveals a barrier to reducing CLABSI, the text below gives guidance to review the approaches, advice, tools, or resources to better implement the CLABSI prevention strategy queried in that question.

Box D.2

CLABSI GUIDE TO PATIENT SAFETY

1. Do you currently collect data related to CLABSI process measures (e.g., central vascular catheters [CVC] prevalence, CVC days) or outcomes (e.g., CLABSI rates)?

☐ Yes   ☐ No

If you answered No, this implies that you do not currently collect CLABSI prevention data such as number of central venous catheters, days of use, or rates of infection. Both unit- and patient-specific data are necessary in order to identify trends in infection rates and measure intervention outcomes. The Centers for Disease Control and Prevention's (CDC's) National Healthcare Safety Network (NHSN) module and Targeted Assessment for Prevention (TAP) strategy tools outline how data can be collected, reported, and used to guide improvement.

For additional tools, resources, and further reading, please visit our Preventing Hospital Infection Resource page at **https://psep.med.umich. edu/phi.html**

See section on Data Collection.

2. Do you routinely report CLABSI-related metrics and data to front-line staff and physicians (e.g., CVC prevalence, CVC days, CLABSI rates)?

☐ Yes   ☐ No

If you answered No, this implies that you do not routinely report CLABSI-related data to front-line staff. Collecting CLABSI-related data is necessary to measure the success of the intervention; however, it is imperative that staff on the front lines are aware of successes and failures. Sharing data is a key method for not only motivating but also engaging staff at all stages of CLABSI prevention work. Access to timely data will also encourage continued changes for sustaining CLABSI reductions.

For additional tools, resources, and further reading, please visit our Preventing Hospital Infection Resource page at **https://psep.med.umich. edu/phi.html**

See section on Infection Prevention Feedback.

3. Does your facility use a standardized CVC insertion tray that includes alcohol-containing chlorhexidine gluconate for skin antisepsis?

☐ Yes   ☐ No

If you answered No, this implies that your facility either does not use a standardized CVC insertion tray or does not use one that contains alcohol-containing chlorhexidine gluconate for skin antisepsis. Many studies have shown that a standardized tray including key equipment (e.g., introducer needle, guidewire, micropuncture kit, antiseptic) helps prevent breaks in sterile procedure when inserting central lines. Use of alcohol-containing chlorhexidine as a skin antiseptic has also been shown to reduce rates of CLABSI in multiple randomized trials and systematic reviews.

For additional tools, resources, and further reading, please visit our Preventing Hospital Infection Resource page at **https://psep.med.umich.edu/phi.html**

See section on Aseptic Insertion.

4. Do nurses have the ability to stop or pause a CVC from being placed if aseptic technique is not being followed by the operator?

☐ Yes   ☐ No

If you answered No, this implies that nurses are not empowered to stop CVC placement if aseptic insertion technique is broken or not being followed. The Michigan Keystone study found drastic reductions when nurses not involved with device placement monitored CVC insertion at bedside and stopped the procedure if maximal sterile barriers and other antisepsis measures were not being followed. Developing a culture of patient safety such as this should be not only encouraged but also appreciated in organizations dedicated to reducing CLABSI.

For additional tools, resources, and further reading, please visit our Preventing Hospital Infection Resource page at **https://psep.med.umich.edu/phi.html**

See section on Nurse Empowerment.

5. Do bedside nurses take initiative and/or have a systematic process to audit and contact physicians to ensure that CVCs are removed when the device is no longer needed?

☐ Yes   ☐ No

If you answered No, this implies that bedside nurses either do not take the initiative or do not have a dedicated process for auditing and/or contacting physicians to ensure that CVCs are removed when no longer clinically necessary. An effective way to prevent CLABSI is to review the necessity of a central line every day and encourage removal of devices that are idle, clinically unnecessary, or no longer clinically indicated. Multidisciplinary rounds and processes that encourage clinicians to continuously reassess central line necessity can have substantial impact on CLABSI reduction.

For additional tools, resources, and further reading, please visit our Preventing Hospital Infection Resource page at **https://psep.med.umich. edu/phi.html**

See section on Catheter Necessity and Removal.

6. Do bedside nurses assess dressing integrity and have the authority to re-place loose, wet, soiled dressings on vascular catheters on a daily basis?

☐ Yes   ☐ No

If you answered No, this implies that bedside nurses either do not assess vascular catheter dressing integrity on a daily basis or do not have the au-thority to replace loose, wet, or soiled dressing when observed. Catheter exit site care is vital in preventing CLABSI. Semitransparent dressings or dressings containing antiseptics are key to preventing bacterial migra-tion from the skin to the bloodstream. Daily rounds that examine cath-eter entry sites, ensure clean and dry dressing, and promptly address exit site issues can prevent maintenance-related infections. A CLABSI preven-tion initiative often relies on a vascular catheter care team that is closely monitoring CVC care and maintenance practices.

For additional tools, resources, and further reading, please visit our Preventing Hospital Infection Resource page at **https://psep.med.umich. edu/phi.html**

See section on Catheter Maintenance.

7. At your facility, do patients and/or families request CVCs such as periph-erally inserted central catheters (PICCs)?

☐ Yes   ☐ No

If you answered Yes, this implies that patients and families often re-quest CVCs in your facility. This is a common and growing trend in the United States as PICCs have become more prevalent. Patients who re-ceived PICCs in the past are likely to request this device again given the comfort associated with lack of needle-sticks for blood draws. However, educating patients on the associated risks is important. Ensuring CVC and PICC use occurs only for appropriate indications is a key step in preventing infection. The Michigan Appropriateness Guide to Intravenous Catheters (MAGIC) is one such document that can help inform this decision.

For additional tools, resources, and further reading, please visit our Preventing Hospital Infection Resource page at **https://psep.med.umich. edu/phi.html**

See section on Patient Education.

8. At your facility are CVCs, such as PICCs, being inserted without an appropriate indication?

☐ Yes   ☐ No or Unknown

If you answered Yes, this implies that CVCs, such as PICCs, are or may be inserted without an appropriate indication in your facility. Ensuring CVC and PICC use occurs only for appropriate indications is a key step in preventing infection. Standardized lists of indications, electronic medical record improvements to facilitate documentation of indication, or working with inserters of CVCs to ensure that the indication is documented can help improve usage of CVCs. MAGIC contains appropriate indications for use of CVCs such as PICCs and tunneled catheters.

For additional tools, resources, and further reading, please visit our Preventing Hospital Infection Resource page at **https://psep.med.umich. edu/phi.html**

See section on Appropriateness.

9. At your facility, do vascular access nurses or operators that insert PICCs have non–central venous catheter options (e.g., ultrasound-guided peripheral intravenous catheters, midline catheters for patients that are known to have difficult venous access?

☐ Yes   ☐ No

If you answered No, this implies that you do not have non–central venous catheter options available for insertion in patients with difficult venous access. It is important to consider investing in peripheral venous access strategies for patients with difficult venous access. Studies showed that such patients often get PICCs for shorter durations or PICCs that could be avoided as non–central venous access is necessary. Obtaining devices that can be inserted under ultrasound guidance such as long peripheral catheters, ultrasound-guided peripheral catheters, or midline catheters can help avoid the need for PICCs in these patients. Training inserters to become comfortable with these devices and developing pathways for use of these devices in difficult intravenous access can help avoid and improve unnecessary PICC use. MAGIC contains indications for use of PICCs and provides guidance on when peripheral devices such as midlines and ultrasound-guided peripheral catheters may be more appropriate than PICCs in specific patient populations.

For additional tools, resources, and further reading, please visit our Preventing Hospital Infection Resource page at **https://psep.med.umich.edu/phi.html**

See section on Non–Central Venous Catheters.

10. Are vascular access nurses empowered to act as "consultants" and insert the most appropriate device for a patient?

☐ Yes   ☐ No

If you answered No, this implies that vascular access nurses are not currently empowered to insert the most appropriate device for a patient. When vascular access nurses or teams act as consultants in assessing a patient to determine their venous anatomy, infusion needs, and available access sites, more appropriate choices about catheter insertion and devices are made. Such "empowered" vascular access teams serve as consultants rather than inserters and can help physicians make more informed choices about vascular catheters. Empowered teams are therefore not "ordered" to place devices, but rather can make recommendations for what device is appropriate given a specific medical indication. Importantly, such teams often have physician champions to support and assist decision-making. These champions often reside in interventional radiology, intensive care, or hospital medicine.

For additional tools, resources, and further reading, please visit our Preventing Hospital Infection Resource page at **https://psep.med.umich.edu/phi.html**

See section on Empowering Vascular Access Teams.

11. Do you have a well-functioning team focusing on CLABSI prevention?

☐ Yes   ☐ No

If you answered No, this implies either that you do not have a team or the one you have does not function well for preventing CLABSI. Developing a partnership between key stakeholders (e.g., intensive care physicians, hospitalists, anesthesiologists, interventional radiologists, or vascular, bedside, and intensive care unit nurses) that insert and care for central lines is key to implementing a prevention initiative. An implementation team in your hospital or unit should consist of stakeholders from these specialties. This team is critical in developing the CLABSI prevention initiative, assisting with implementation, and monitoring infection rates. Key responsibilities of this team are education, data collection, and evaluation. More than one role may be filled by a single member, and some roles may be short or long term.

For additional tools, resources, and further reading, please visit our Preventing Hospital Infection Resource page at **https://psep.med.umich.edu/phi.html**

See section on Identifying Stakeholders.

12. Do you have a team leader with dedicated time to coordinate CLABSI prevention activities?

☐ Yes   ☐ No

If you answered No, this implies either that you do not have a team leader or that the one you have does not have appropriate time for CLABSI prevention. A team leader is responsible for coordinating the CLABSI prevention efforts, such as data collection, organizing reports, presenting outcomes, and tracking progress. They are responsible for keeping the improvement moving forward and for coordinating moving pieces between stakeholders. Because a team leader likely has multiple responsibilities aside from the intervention, there may not be enough time devoted to prevention efforts. Creating dedicated time for the initiative is imperative to its success.

For additional tools, resources, and further reading, please visit our Preventing Hospital Infection Resource page at **https://psep.med.umich.edu/phi.html**

See section on Identifying a Team Leader.

13. Do you have an effective nurse champion for your CLABSI prevention activities?

☐ Yes   ☐ No

If you answered No, this implies either that you do not have a nurse champion or that the one you have is not effective when it comes to CLABSI prevention activities. Buy-in from nurses is critical to a CLABSI prevention initiative as they play key roles in CVC insertion, are responsible for care and maintenance, and are members of multidisciplinary teams that review catheter necessity on a daily basis.

The nurse champion is responsible for engaging nursing staff in CLABSI prevention efforts and working to integrate practices into nurses' daily workflow. A nurse champion is important for both problem-solving as challenges arise and modeling excitement for infection prevention efforts. Through the nurse champion, a critical link is made between the multidisciplinary team and front-line clinicians, supplying actionable data for change.

For additional tools, resources, and further reading, please visit our Preventing Hospital Infection Resource page at **https://psep.med.umich.edu/phi.html**

See section on Identifying a Nurse Champion.

14. Do you have an effective physician champion for CLABSI prevention activities?

☐ Yes   ☐ No

If you answered No, this implies either that you do not have a physician champion for your CLABSI prevention activities or that the one you have is not effective. Having a respected physician leader is an important part of the cultural aspect of overcoming CLABSI. An ideal physician champion is either involved in the insertion of CVCs (e.g., critical care, surgery, interventional radiologists) or in the ordering of devices (e.g., hospitalists). An effective physician champion is responsible for problem solving as challenges arise and modeling excitement toward the CLABSI prevention efforts. Through the physician champion, a critical link is made between the multidisciplinary team and front-line clinicians, supplying actionable data for change.

For additional tools, resources, and further reading, please visit our Preventing Hospital Infection Resource page at **https://psep.med.umich.edu/phi.html**

See section on Identifying a Physician Champion.

15. Does senior leadership support your CLABSI prevention activities?

☐ Yes   ☐ No

If you answered No, this implies that you do not have the support of senior leadership for your CLABSI prevention activities. Prevention initiatives are costly and often require approval from managerial staff in departments, such as medical executive leadership, purchasing, and accounts. The Michigan Keystone study required senior leadership presence during CLABSI meetings, which benefitted the initiative, as data and action items could be reviewed and discussed with the multidisciplinary team. These meetings help ensure buy-in from those that may not have clinical roles but make decisions regarding supplies and purchases. Having a member of the hospital executive leadership team oversee the initiative also reminds hospital staff of the importance of the initiative.

For additional tools, resources, and further reading, please visit our Preventing Hospital Infection Resource page at **https://psep.med.umich.edu/phi.html**

See section on Senior Leadership Support.

Source: Updated from Saint et al.[15]

To accurately assess the organization's *Clostridioides difficile* infection (CDI) prevention efforts, it is recommended that:

1. The individual or team working on CDI prevention at the hospital or unit level complete the CDI GPS assessment. This can be done independently or as a group.
2. The responses are reviewed as a team as a means to uncover strengths and barriers to reducing CDI.
3. For each question, if a response is chosen that reveals a barrier to reducing CDI, the text below gives guidance to review the approaches, advice, tools, or resources to better implement the CDI prevention strategy queried in that question.

Box D.3

CDI Guide to Patient Safety

1. Do you currently collect data related to CDI (e.g., incidence, prevalence, compliance with prevention practices) in the unit(s) or populations in which you are intervening to reduce infection?

☐ Yes   ☐ No

If you answered No, this implies that you do not currently collect CDI-related data. Collection and analysis of data on your CDI prevention activities are critical to ensure continued success. Outcome data enables you to monitor the success of your CDI prevention initiatives and allows teams to see how they are doing in their prevention efforts to compare it to other units and hospitals. Process measures, such as hand hygiene compliance rates and the use of high-risk antibiotics, ensure that process interventions are being effectively implemented and highlight areas that require continued improvement.

For additional tools, resources, and further reading, please visit our Preventing Hospital Infection Resource page at **https://psep.med.umich.edu/phi.html**

See section on Data Collection.

2. Do you routinely report CDI-related metrics and data to front-line staff and physicians (e.g., incidence, prevalence, compliance with prevention practices, etc.)?

☐ Yes   ☐ No

If you answered No, this implies that you do not routinely report CDI-related data to front-line staff. Staff awareness of CDI-related data is an important part of quality improvement. Data transparency can help motivate and engage staff at all stages of the initiative and encourage them to continue the changes, promoting sustainability. Reporting data to staff improves motivation and engagement. Provide data from your own hospital, as well as data from comparable hospitals and national aggregates. A CDI scorecard can be a great way to display and communicate data to both front-line staff and senior leaders.

For additional tools, resources, and further reading, please visit our Preventing Hospital Infection Resource page at **https://psep.med.umich.edu/phi.html**

See section on Infection Prevention Feedback.

3. Have you educated clinicians regarding when to order CDI testing?

☐ Yes   ☐ No

If you answered No, this implies that clinicians are not educated regarding when it is appropriate to order CDI testing. *Clostridioides difficile* infection is a clinical diagnosis, and while lab tests help support a clinical suspicion, they should not be taken out of the clinical context. Clinicians must be informed of high *C. difficile* colonization rates to illustrate that indiscriminate testing will lead to false-positive results.

For additional tools, resources, and further reading, please visit our Preventing Hospital Infection Resource page at **https://psep.med.umich.edu/phi.html**

See section Education on Testing.

4. Does your laboratory reject formed stools submitted for CDI testing?

☐ Yes   ☐ No

If you answered No, this implies that your laboratory does not reject formed stools submitted for CDI testing. Remember that *C. difficile* infection is a clinical diagnosis, and while lab tests help support a clinical suspicion, they should not be taken out of the clinical context. To limit inappropriate testing, it is recommended that clinical laboratories set a threshold on the type of stool that is acceptable for *C. difficile* testing.

For additional tools, resources, and further reading, please visit our Preventing Hospital Infection Resource page at **https://psep.med.umich.edu/phi.html**

See section on Appropriate Testing.

5. Do you have a hospital antibiotic stewardship team that includes a physician and pharmacist?

☐ Yes   ☐ No

If you answered No, this implies that you do not have at least one physician and one pharmacist engaged on your hospital's antibiotic stewardship team. The single highest risk factor for developing CDI is inappropriate and avoidable exposure to antibiotics; therefore, a successful CDI prevention initiative requires collaboration with both physicians and pharmacists. These team members may help bring the initiative to the other physicians and pharmacists, encourage engagement, and be a part of problem-solving when resistance occurs. The CDC has published guidance on elements for hospitals, including guidance for small and critical access facilities and resource-limited settings.

For additional tools, resources, and further reading, please visit our Preventing Hospital Infection Resource page at **https://psep.med.umich.edu/phi.html**

See section on Antibiotic Stewardship Teams.

6. Do you have antibiotic stewardship teams that include a physician and pharmacist for ambulatory (outpatient) care and/or nursing homes associated with your hospital?

☐ Yes   ☐ No

If you answered No, this implies that you do not have at least one physician and/or one pharmacist engaged on your antibiotic stewardship team(s) dedicated to the ambulatory or nursing home setting. The single highest risk factor for developing CDI is inappropriate and avoidable exposure to antibiotics; therefore, a successful CDI prevention initiative requires collaboration with both physicians and pharmacists. These team members may help bring the initiative to the other physicians and pharmacists, encourage engagement, and be a part of problem-solving when resistance occurs. The CDC has published guidance on elements for ambulatory stewardship programs in ambulatory/outpatient care and nursing home settings.

For additional tools, resources, and further reading, please visit our Preventing Hospital Infection Resource page at **https://psep.med.umich.edu/phi.html**

See section on Antibiotic Stewardship Teams.

7. Do you conduct audits and provide feedback on the effectiveness of environmental cleaning?

☐ Yes   ☐ No

If you answered No, this implies that you do not conduct audits or provide feedback to staff on the effectiveness of environmental cleaning. *Clostridioides difficile* bacteria or bacterial spores can contaminate the patient or their environment and then be passed on to other patients via healthcare personnel or shared equipment or to the next occupant of the patient room. Hospitals and units need to ensure that environmental cleaning and disinfection are effectively decontaminating patient rooms and equipment in order to prevent CDI transmission.

For additional tools, resources, and further reading, please visit our Preventing Hospital Infection Resource page at **https://psep.med.umich.edu/phi.html**

See section on Environmental Cleaning.

8. Is staff empowered to speak up and remind colleagues about proper hand hygiene and personal protective equipment use?

☐ Yes   ☐ No

If you answered No, this implies that staff are not empowered to speak up to remind colleagues to perform proper hand hygiene and use personal protective equipment. Preventing CDI relies on preventing its transmission. Staff should be encouraged to remind colleagues about proper protective measures. A facility-wide reminder phrase may be used to get everyone on the same page and keep reminders from feeling punitive.

For additional tools, resources, and further reading, please visit our Preventing Hospital Infection Resource page at **https://psep.med.umich.edu/phi.html**

See section on Staff Empowerment.

9. Do you have a well-functioning team focusing on CDI prevention?

☐ Yes   ☐ No

If you answered No, this implies either that you do not have a team or work group or the one you have does not function well. Identifying an implementation team at your site is key to a successful intervention. Among the responsibilities of this team are education, data collection, and evaluation. Team members may fill more than one role, and roles may be short term or long term.

For additional tools, resources, and further reading, please visit our Preventing Hospital Infection Resource page at **https://psep.med.umich.edu/phi.html**

See section on Identifying a Team.

10. Do you have a team leader with dedicated time to coordinate CDI prevention activities?

☐ Yes   ☐ No

If you answered No, this implies either that you do not have a team leader or that the one you have does not have appropriate time for the initiative. The team leader is responsible for many tasks, including coordinating and facilitating team meetings, communication, and overseeing team members. It is imperative that she or he has dedicated time to commit to the project.

For additional tools, resources, and further reading, please visit our Preventing Hospital Infection Resource page at **https://psep.med.umich.edu/phi.html**

See section on Identifying a Team Leader.

11. Do you have an effective physician champion for CDI prevention activities?

☐ Yes   ☐ No

If you answered No, this implies either that you do not have a physician champion or that the one you have is not effective. The physician champion is responsible for engaging physicians in CDI prevention efforts and coordinating prevention efforts that require physician support. An ideal physician champion is well respected, trusted by peers, supportive of safety, and an agent of change.

For additional tools, resources, and further reading, please visit our Preventing Hospital Infection Resource page at **https://psep.med.umich.edu/phi.html**

See section on Identifying a Physician Champion.

12. Does senior leadership support your CDI prevention activities?

☐ Yes   ☐ No

If you answered No, this implies that you do not have the support of senior leadership. Having the support of leadership is important for making immediate and lasting change with a prevention initiative. Having a member of the hospital executive leadership team oversee the initiative also informs the hospital of the importance of the initiative.

For additional tools, resources, and further reading, please visit our Preventing Hospital Infection Resource page at **https://psep.med.umich.edu/phi.html**

See section on Senior Leadership Support.

Source: Updated from Saint et al.[1,6]

Michigan Appropriateness Guide for Intravenous
Catheters (MAGIC) Criteria

Box E.1

GUIDE FOR PICC USE

Appropriate indications for PICC use

Delivery of peripherally compatible infusates when the proposed
duration of such use is ≥ 6 d*

Delivery of non–peripherally compatible infusates (e.g., irritants or
vesicants), regardless of proposed duration of use

Delivery of cyclical or episodic chemotherapy that can be administered
through a peripheral vein in patients with active cancer, provided
that the proposed duration of such treatment is ≥ 3 months†

Invasive hemodynamic monitoring or requirement to obtain
central venous access in a critically ill patient, provided the
proposed duration of such use is ≥ 15 days‡

Frequent phlebotomy (every 8 hours) in a hospitalized patient,
provided that the proposed duration of such use is ≥ 6 days

Intermittent infusions or infrequent phlebotomy in patients with
poor/difficult peripheral venous access, provided that the
proposed duration of such use is ≥ 6 days§

For infusions or palliative treatment during end-of-life care||

Delivery of peripherally compatible infusates for patients residing
in skilled nursing facilities or transitional from hospital to home,
provided that the proposed duration of such use is ≥ 15 days¶

Inappropriate indications for PICC use

Placement for any indication other than infusion of non–
   peripherally compatible infusates (e.g., irritants or vesicants)
   when the proposed duration of use is ≤ 5 days

Placement in a patient with active cancer for cyclical chemotherapy
   that can be administered through a peripheral vein when
   the proposed duration of such treatment is ≤ 3 months and
   peripheral veins are available

Placement in a patient with Stage 3b or greater chronic kidney disease
   (estimated glomerular filtration rate ≤ 44 mL/min) or in patients
   currently receiving renal replacement therapy via any modality

Insertion for nonfrequent phlebotomy if the proposed duration of
   such use is ≤ 5 days

Patient or family request in a patient who is not actively dying or
   in hospice, for comfort in obtaining daily blood samples for
   laboratory analysis

Medical or nursing provider request in the absence of other
   appropriate criteria for PICC use

Reprinted with permission from Annals of Internal Medicine.[1]

PICC = peripherally inserted central catheter.

* Use of ultrasonography-guided peripheral intravenous catheters or midlines is preferred over use of PICCs for infusion of peripherally compatible infusates up to 14 d. In patients with poor peripheral venous access, use of ultrasonography-guided peripheral intravenous catheters and midlines is also preferred over use of PICCS.

† In patients with cancer, the risk for thrombosis associated with PICCs may outweigh benefits. Patients who are scheduled to receive multiple cycles of peripherally compatible chemotherapy for durations <3 mo should do so via peripheral intravenous catheters with each infusion.

‡ Use of nontunneled central venous catheters is preferred over use of PICCs for central venous access or invasive hemodynamic monitoring <14 d and in patients with documented hemody-namic instability where urgent venous access is necessary.

§ Use of ultrasonography-guided peripheral intravenous catheters or midlines is preferred over use of PICCs for patients with poor/difficult peripheral venous access.

|| Placement of a PICC in a terminally ill patient is appropriate if it facilitates comfort goals of care. PICCs may be left in place in such patients to attain similar goals.

¶ Use of PICCs for home-based infusions or in skilled nursing facilities (where resources are limited) is inappropriate for short-term durations (<14 d). In such settings, use of peripheral intravenous catheters or midlines was rated as appropriate.

Device Type	Proposed Duration of Infusion			
	≤5 d	6–14 d	15–30 d	≥31 d
Peripheral IV catheter	*No preference between peripheral IV and US-guided peripheral IV catheters for use ≤5 d*			
US-guided peripheral IV catheter	*US-guided peripheral IV catheter preferred to peripheral IV catheter if proposed duration 6–14 d*			
Nontunneled/ acute central venous catheter	*Central venous catheters preferred in critically ill patients or if hemodynamic monitoring is needed for 6–14 d*			
Midline catheter	*Midline catheter preferred to PICC if proposed duration ≤14 d*			
PICC		*PICC preferred to midline catheter if proposed duration of infusion ≥15 d*		
Tunneled catheter				*PICC preferred to tunneled catheter and ports for infusions 15–30 d*
Port				

Appropriate Neutral Inappropriate Disagreement

Figure E.1 Venous access device recommendations for infusion of *peripherally compatible* infusates. IV, intravenous; PICC, peripherally inserted central catheter; US, ultrasound. (Reprinted with permission from *Annals of Internal Medicine*.[1])

Device Type	Proposed Duration of Infusion			
	≤5 d	6–14 d	15–30 d	≥31 d
Peripheral IV catheter				
US-guided peripheral IV catheter				
Nontunneled/ acute central venous catheter	*Central venous catheter preferred in critically ill patients or if hemodynamic monitoring is needed for 6–14 days*			
Midline catheter				
PICC	*PICCs rated as appropriate at all proposed durations of infusion*			
Tunneled catheter		*Tunneled catheter neutral for use ≥15 d*	*No preference between tunneled catheter and PICC for proposed durations ≥15 d*	
Port				*No preference among port, tunneled catheter or PICC for ≥31 d*

Appropriate Neutral Inappropriate Disagreement

Figure E.2 Venous access device recommendations for infusion of *non–peripherally compatible* infusates. IV, intravenous; PICC, peripherally inserted central catheter; US, ultrasound. (Reprinted with permission from *Annals of Internal Medicine*.[1])

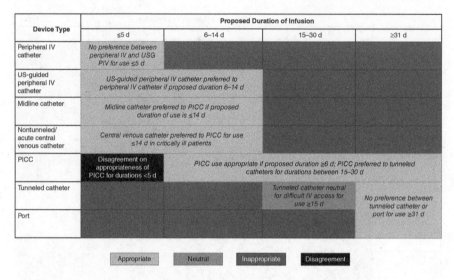

Figure E.3 Venous access device recommendations for patients with difficult venous access. IV, intravenous; PICC, peripherally inserted central catheter; US, ultrasound. (Reprinted with permission from *Annals of Internal Medicine*.[1])

Device Type	Proposed Duration of Infusion			
	≤5 d	6–14 d	15–30 d	≥31 d
Peripheral IV catheter	No preference between peripheral IV and US-guided peripheral IV catheter for use ≤5 d			
US-guided peripheral IV catheter	US-guided peripheral IV catheter preferred if venous access difficult			
Midline catheter	Midline catheter preferred to PICCs if proposed duration is ≤14 d		Midline catheter neutral for frequent phlebotomy at this duration	
Nontunneled/ acute central venous catheter	Central venous catheter preferred to PICC for use ≤14 d in critically ill patients			
PICC	Disagreement on appropriateness of PICC for durations <5 d	PICC use appropriate if proposed duration ≥6 d; PICC preferred to tunneled catheter for durations between 15–30 d		
Tunneled catheter			Tunneled catheter neutral for difficult intravenous access for use ≥15 d	
Port	Ports inappropriate for frequent phlebotomy, regardless of proposed duration of use			

Appropriate Neutral Inappropriate Disagreement

Figure E.4 Venous access device recommendations for patients who require frequent phlebotomy. IV, intravenous; PICC, peripherally inserted central catheter; US, ultrasound. (Modified with permission from *Annals of Internal Medicine*.[1])

CHAPTER 1: AN EFFECTIVE STRATEGY TO COMBAT HOSPITAL INFECTIONS

1. Harbarth S, Sax H, Gastmeier P. The preventable proportion of nosocomial infections: an overview of published reports. J Hosp Infect. 2003;54:258–266; quiz 321.
2. Umscheid CA, Mitchell MD, Doshi JA, Agarwal R, Williams K, Brennan PJ. Estimating the proportion of healthcare-associated infections that are reasonably preventable and the related mortality and costs. Infect Control Hosp Epidemiol. 2011;32:101–114.
3. Magill SS, O'Leary E, Janelle SJ, et al. Changes in prevalence of health care-associated infections in US hospitals. N Engl J Med. 2018;379:1732–1744.
4. Saint S, Greene MT, Krein SL, et al. A program to prevent catheter-associated urinary tract infection in acute care. N Engl J Med. 2016;374:2111–2119.
5. Schreiber PW, Sax H, Wolfensberger A, Clack L, Kuster SP, Swissnoso. The preventable proportion of healthcare-associated infections 2005–2016: systematic review and meta-analysis. Infect Control Hosp Epidemiol. 2018;39:1277–1295.
6. Patel PK, Gupta A, Vaughn VM, Mann JD, Ameling JM, Meddings J. Review of strategies to reduce central line-associated bloodstream infection (CLABSI) and catheter-associated urinary tract infection (CAUTI) in adult ICUs. J Hosp Med. 2018;13:105–116.
7. 2018 National and state healthcare-associated infections progress report. Accessed July 24, 2020, at https://www.cdc.gov/hai/data/portal/progress-report.html
8. Patel PK, Greene MT, Jones K, et al. Quantitative results of a national intervention to prevent central line-associated bloodstream infection: a pre-post observational study. Ann Intern Med. 2019;171:S23–S29.
9. Meddings J, Manojlovich M, Ameling JM, et al. Quantitative results of a national intervention to prevent hospital-acquired catheter-associated urinary tract infection: a pre-post observational study. Ann Intern Med. 2019;171:S38–S44.

10. Meddings J, Greene MT, Ratz D, et al. Multistate programme to reduce catheter-associated infections in intensive care units with elevated infection rates. BMJ Qual Saf. 2020;29:418–429.

11. Saint S, Greene MT, Fowler KE, et al. What US hospitals are currently doing to prevent common device-associated infections: results from a national survey. BMJ Qual Saf. 2019;28:741–749.

12. Dubberke ER, Rohde JM, Saint S, et al. Quantitative results of a national intervention to prevent *Clostridioides difficile* infection: a pre-post observational study. Ann Intern Med. 2019;171:S52–S58.

13. Calfee DP, Davila S, Chopra V, et al. Quantitative results of a national intervention to prevent hospital-onset methicillin-resistant *Staphylococcus aureus* bloodstream infection: a pre-post observational study. Ann Intern Med. 2019;171:S66–S72.

14. National action plan to prevent health-care associated infections: road map to elimination. Accessed July 24, 2020, at https://health.gov/hcq/prevent-hai-action-plan.asp

15. Medicare program; changes to the hospital inpatient prospective payment systems and fiscal year 2008 rates. Federal Register. 2007;72(162):47129–48175.

16. Hospital-acquired conditions (Present on Admission Indicator). Centers for Medicare & Medicaid Services. Accessed July 24, 2020, at https://www.cms.gov/Medicare/Medicare-Fee-for-Service-Payment/HospitalAcqCond/index.html

17. Hospital-Acquired Condition Reduction Program (HACRP). Centers for Medicare & Medicaid Services. Accessed July 24, 2020, at https://www.cms.gov/medicare/medicare-fee-for-service-payment/acuteinpatientpps/hac-reduction-program.html

18. CMS requirements. Centers for Disease Control and Prevention. Accessed July 24, 2020, at https://www.cdc.gov/nhsn/cms/index.html

19. Meddings J, Rogers MAM, Macy M, Saint S. Systematic review and meta-analysis: reminder systems to reduce catheter-associated urinary tract infections and urinary catheter use in hospitalized patients. Clin Infect Dis. 2010;51:550–560.

20. Meddings J, Rogers MA, Krein SL, Fakih MG, Olmsted RN, Saint S. Reducing unnecessary urinary catheter use and other strategies to prevent catheter-associated urinary tract infection: an integrative review. BMJ Qual Saf. 2014;23:277–289.

21. Meddings J, Saint S, Fowler KE, et al. The Ann Arbor Criteria for Appropriate Urinary Catheter Use in Hospitalized Medical Patients: Results Obtained by Using the RAND/UCLA Appropriateness Method. Ann Intern Med. 2015;162:S1–S34.

22. Meddings J, Skolarus TA, Fowler KE, et al. Michigan Appropriate Perioperative (MAP) criteria for urinary catheter use in common general and orthopaedic surgeries: results obtained using the RAND/UCLA Appropriateness Method. BMJ Qual Saf. 2019;28:56–66.

23. Chopra V, Flanders SA, Saint S, et al. The Michigan Appropriateness Guide for Intravenous Catheters (MAGIC): Results from a Multispecialty Panel Using the RAND/UCLA. Ann Intern Med. 2015;163:S1–S40.

24. *Candida auris.* Centers for Disease Control and Prevention 2019. Accessed July 24, 2020, at https://www.cdc.gov/fungal/candida-auris/index.html

CHAPTER 2: COMMITTING TO AN INFECTION PREVENTION INITIATIVE

1. Hospital compare: complications & deaths. US Centers for Medicare & Medicaid Services. Accessed July 24, 2020, at https://www.medicare.gov/hospitalcompare/About/Complications.html

2. Changing health care. Joint Commission Center for Transforming Healthcare. Accessed July 24, 2020, at https://www.centerfortransforminghealthcare.org/

3. High reliability. Agency for Healthcare Research and Quality. Accessed July 24, 2020, at https://psnet.ahrq.gov/primer/high-reliability

4. Improving the reliability of health care. Institute for Healthcare Improvement, 2004. Accessed July 24, 2020, at http://www.ihi.org/resources/Pages/IHIWhitePapers/ImprovingtheReliabilityofHealthCare.aspx

5. A framework for safe, reliable, and effective care. Institute for Healthcare Improvement and Safe & Reliable Healthcare, 2017. Accessed July 24, 2020, at http://www.ihi.org/resources/Pages/IHIWhitePapers/Framework-Safe-Reliable-Effective-Care.aspx

6. Hospital-acquired conditions. Centers for Medicare & Medicaid Services. Accessed July 24, 2020, at https://www.cms.gov/Medicare/Medicare-Fee-for-Service-Payment/HospitalAcqCond/Hospital-Acquired_Conditions

7. Saint S, Meddings JA, Calfee D, Kowalski CP, Krein SL. Catheter-associated urinary tract infection and the Medicare rule changes. Ann Intern Med. 2009;150:877–884.

8. McNair PD, Luft HS, Bindman AB. Medicare's policy not to pay for treating hospital-acquired conditions: the impact. Health Aff (Millwood). 2009;28:1485–1493.

9. Lee GM, Kleinman K, Soumerai SB, et al. Effect of nonpayment for preventable infections in US hospitals. N Engl J Med. 2012;367:1428–1437.

10. Kawai AT, Calderwood MS, Jin R, et al. Impact of the Centers for Medicare and Medicaid Services hospital-acquired conditions policy on billing rates for 2 targeted healthcare-associated infections. Infect Control Hosp Epidemiol. 2015;36:871–877.

11. Meddings J, Saint S, McMahon LF Jr. Hospital-acquired catheter-associated urinary tract infection: documentation and coding issues may reduce financial impact of Medicare's new payment policy. Infect Control Hosp Epidemiol. 2010;31:627–633.

12. Lee GM, Hartmann CW, Graham D, et al. Perceived impact of the Medicare policy to adjust payment for health care-associated infections. Am J Infect Control. 2012;40:314–319.

13. Meddings JA, Reichert H, Rogers MA, Saint S, Stephansky J, McMahon LF. Effect of nonpayment for hospital-acquired, catheter-associated urinary tract infection: a statewide analysis. Ann Intern Med. 2012 Sep 4;157(5):305–12. doi: 10.7326/0003-4819-157-5-201209040-00003.

14. National Healthcare Safety Network (NHSN) patient safety component manual. Centers for Disease Control and Prevention 2020. Accessed July 24, 2020, at https://www.cdc.gov/nhsn/pdfs/pscmanual/pcsmanual_current.pdf

15. The NHSN Standardized Infection Ratio (SIR). Centers for Disease Control and Prevention, 2019. Accessed July 24, 2020, at https://www.cdc.gov/nhsn/pdfs/ps-analysis-resources/nhsn-sir-guide.pdf

16. Hospital-Acquired Condition Reduction Program (HACRP). Centers for Medicare & Medicaid Services. Accessed July 24, 2020, at https://www.cms.gov/medicare/medicare-fee-for-service-payment/acuteinpatientpps/hac-reduction-program.html

17. The Hospital Value-Based Purchasing (VBP) program. Accessed July 24, 2020, at https://www.cms.gov/Medicare/Quality-Initiatives-Patient-Assessment-Instruments/Value-Based-Programs/HVBP/Hospital-Value-Based-Purchasing

18. Meddings J, McMahon LF Jr. Web exclusives. Annals for hospitalists inpatient notes—legislating quality to prevent infection—a primer for hospitalists. Ann Intern Med. 2017;166:HO2–HO3.

19. Data summary of HAIs in the US: assessing progress 2006–2016. Centers for Disease Control and Prevention, 2017. Accessed July 24, 2020, at https://www.cdc.gov/hai/data/archive/data-summary-assessing-progress.html

20. HAI [Healthcare-Associated Infection] data. Centers for Disease Control and Prevention, 2018. Accessed July 24, 2020, at https://www.cdc.gov/hai/data/index.html

21. Saving lives and saving money: hospital-acquired conditions update. Agency for Healthcare Research & Quality, 2015. Accessed July 24, 2020, at https://www.ahrq.gov/hai/pfp/interimhacrate2014.html

22. Magill SS, O'Leary E, Janelle SJ, et al. Changes in prevalence of health care-associated infections in US hospitals. N Engl J Med. 2018;379:1732–1744.

23. Magid B, Murphy C, Lankiewicz J, Lawandi N, Poulton A. Pricing for safety and quality in healthcare: a discussion paper. Infect Dis Health. 2018;23:49–53.

24. Addendum to the National Health Reform Agreement: revised public hospital arrangements (Schedule 1). Council on Federal Financial Regulations (Australia), 2017. Accessed July 24, 2020, at http://www.federalfinancialrelations.gov.au/content/npa/health/other/Addendum_to_the_National_Health_Reform.pdf

25. The NHS payment system: evolving policy and emerging evidence. Nuffield Trust, 2014. Accessed July 24, 2020, at https://www.nuffieldtrust.org.uk/files/2017-01/2014-nhs-payment-research-report-web-final.pdf

26. Aligning outcomes and spending: Canadian experiences with value-based healthcare. Canadian Foundation for Healthcare Improvement, 2018. Accessed July 24, 2020, at https://www.cfhi-fcass.ca/sf-docs/default-source/documents/health-system-transformation/vbhc-executive-brief-e.pdf?sfvrsn=c884ab44_2

27. Saint S, Olmsted RN, Fakih MG, et al. Translating health care-associated urinary tract infection prevention research into practice via the bladder bundle. Jt Comm J Qual Patient Saf. 2009;35:449–455.

28. With money at risk, hospitals push staff to wash hands. New York Times. 2013, May 29. Accessed July 24, 2020, at https://www.nytimes.com/2013/05/29/nyregion/hospitals-struggle-to-get-workers-to-wash-their-hands.html

CHAPTER 3: TYPES OF INTERVENTIONS: CATHETER-ASSOCIATED

URINARY TRACT INFECTION

1. Erasmus V, Daha TJ, Brug H, et al. Systematic review of studies on compliance with hand hygiene guidelines in hospital care. Infect Control Hosp Epidemiol. 2010;31:283–294.

2. Saint S, Lipsky BA, Baker PD, McDonald LL, Ossenkop K. Urinary catheters: what type do men and their nurses prefer? J Am Geriatr Soc. 1999;47:1453–1457.

3. Nicolle LE. Catheter associated urinary tract infections. Antimicrob Resist Infect Control 2014;3:23.

4. Manojlovich M, Saint S, Meddings J, et al. Indwelling urinary catheter insertion practices in the emergency department: an observational study. Infect Control Hosp Epidemiol. 2016;37:117–119.

5. The RAND/UCLA Appropriateness Method user's manual. Directorate General XII, European Commission, 2001. Accessed July 24, 2020, at https://www.rand.org/content/dam/rand/pubs/monograph_reports/2011/MR1269.pdf

6. Skolarus TA, Dauw CA, Fowler KE, Mann JD, Bernstein SJ, Meddings J. Catheter management after benign transurethral prostate surgery: RAND/UCLA Appropriateness Criteria. Am J Manag Care. 2019;25:e366–e372.

7. Gray M, Skinner C, Kaler W. External collection devices as an alternative to the indwelling urinary catheter: evidence-based review and expert clinical panel deliberations. J Wound Ostomy Continence Nurs. 2016;43:301–307.

8. Dublynn T, Episcopia B. Female external catheter use: a new bundle element to reduce CAUTI. Am J Infect Control. 2019;47:S39–S40.

9. Beeson T, Davis C. Urinary management with an external female collection device. J Wound Ostomy Continence Nurs. 2018;45:187–189.

10. Meddings J, Saint S, Fowler KE, et al. The Ann Arbor Criteria for Appropriate Urinary Catheter Use in Hospitalized Medical Patients: Results Obtained by Using the RAND/UCLA Appropriateness Method. Ann Intern Med. 2015;162:S1–S34.

11. Cornia PB, Amory JK, Fraser S, Saint S, Lipsky BA. Computer-based order entry decreases duration of indwelling urinary catheterization in hospitalized patients. Am J Med. 2003;114:404–407.

12. Saint S, Kaufman SR, Thompson M, Rogers MA, Chenoweth CE. A reminder reduces urinary catheterization in hospitalized patients. Jt Comm J Qual Patient Saf. 2005;31:455–462.

13. Gould CV, Umscheid CA, Agarwal RK, Kuntz G, Pegues DA. Healthcare Infection Control Practices Advisory Committee (HICPAC). Guideline for prevention of catheter-associated urinary tract infections 2009. Infect Control Hosp Epidemiol. 2010;31:319–326.

14. Meddings J, Rogers MA, Krein SL, Fakih MG, Olmsted RN, Saint S. Reducing unnecessary urinary catheter use and other strategies to prevent catheter-associated urinary tract infection: an integrative review. BMJ Qual Saf. 2014;23:277–289.

15. Patel PK, Gupta A, Vaughn VM, Mann JD, Ameling JM, Meddings J. Review of strategies to reduce central line-associated bloodstream infection (CLABSI) and catheter-associated urinary tract infection (CAUTI) in adult ICUs. J Hosp Med. 2018;13:105–116.

16. Popovich KJ, Calfee DP, Patel PK, et al. The Centers for Disease Control and Prevention STRIVE initiative: construction of a national program to reduce health care-associated infections at the local level. Ann Intern Med. 2019;171:S2–S6.

17. Meddings J, Manojlovich M, Fowler KE, et al. A tiered approach for preventing catheter-associated urinary tract infection. Ann Intern Med. 2019;171:S30–S37.

18. Saint S, Meddings J, Fowler KE, et al. The guide to patient safety for health care-associated infections. Ann Intern Med. 2019;171:S7–S9.

19. Saint S, Gaies E, Fowler KE, Harrod M, Krein SL. Introducing a catheter-associated urinary tract infection (CAUTI) prevention guide to patient safety (GPS). Am J Infect Control. 2014;42:548–550.

{}{}{}{}{}

20. Fletcher KE, Tyszka JT, Harrod M, Fowler KE, Saint S, Krein SL. Qualitative validation of the CAUTI Guide to Patient Safety assessment tool. Am J Infect Control. 2016;44:1102–1109.

21. Meddings J, Manojlovich M, Ameling JM, et al. Quantitative results of a national intervention to prevent hospital-acquired catheter-associated urinary tract infection: a pre-post observational study. Ann Intern Med. 2019;171:S38–S44.

22. Fowler KE, Forman J, Ameling JM, et al. Qualitative assessment of a state partner-facilitated health care-associated infection prevention national collaborative. Ann Intern Med. 2019;171:S75–S80.

23. Smith GC, Pell JP. Parachute use to prevent death and major trauma related to gravitational challenge: systematic review of randomised controlled trials. BMJ. 2003;327:1459–1461.

24. Yeh RW, Valsdottir LR, Yeh MW, et al. Parachute use to prevent death and major trauma when jumping from aircraft: randomized controlled trial. BMJ. 2018;363:k5094.

CHAPTER 4: TYPES OF INTERVENTIONS: CENTRAL LINE–ASSOCIATED BLOODSTREAM INFECTION

1. Simonov M, Pittiruti M, Rickard CM, Chopra V. Navigating venous access: a guide for hospitalists. J Hosp Med. 2015;10:471–478.

2. Vital signs: central line-associated blood stream infections—United States, 2001, 2008, and 2009. Centers for Disease Control and Prevention, 2011. Accessed July 24, 2020, at https://www.cdc.gov/mmwr/preview/mmwrhtml/mm6008a4.htm

3. Magill SS, O'Leary E, Janelle SJ, et al. Changes in prevalence of health care-associated infections in US hospitals. N Engl J Med. 2018;379:1732–1744.

4. Pronovost P, Needham D, Berenholtz S, et al. An intervention to decrease catheter-related bloodstream infections in the ICU. N Engl J Med. 2006;355:2725–2732.

5. Render ML, Hasselbeck R, Freyberg RW, et al. Reduction of central line infections in Veterans Administration intensive care units: an observational cohort using a central infrastructure to support learning and improvement. BMJ Qual Saf. 2011;20:725–732.

6. Climo M, Diekema D, Warren DK, et al. Prevalence of the use of central venous access devices within and outside of the intensive care unit: results of a survey among hospitals in the prevention epicenter program of the Centers for Disease Control and Prevention. Infect Control Hosp Epidemiol. 2003;24:942–945.

7. Zingg W, Sandoz L, Inan C, et al. Hospital-wide survey of the use of central venous catheters. J Hosp Infect. 2011;77:304–308.

8. Marschall J, Leone C, Jones M, Nihill D, Fraser VJ, Warren DK. Catheter-associated bloodstream infections in general medical patients outside the intensive care unit: a surveillance study. Infect Control Hosp Epidemiol. 2007;28:905–909.

9. Chopra V, Flanders SA, Saint S. The problem with peripherally inserted central catheters. JAMA. 2012;308:1527–1528.

10. Pikwer A, Akeson J, Lindgren S. Complications associated with peripheral or central routes for central venous cannulation. Anaesthesia. 2012;67:65–71.

11. Chopra V, O'Horo JC, Rogers MA, Maki DG, Safdar N. The risk of bloodstream infection associated with peripherally inserted central catheters compared with central venous catheters in adults: a systematic review and meta-analysis. Infect Control Hosp Epidemiol. 2013;34:908–918.

12. Al Raiy B, Fakih MG, Bryan-Nomides N, et al. Peripherally inserted central venous catheters in the acute care setting: a safe alternative to high-risk short-term central venous catheters. Am J Infect Control. 2010;38:149–153.

13. Chopra V, Anand S, Hickner A, et al. Risk of venous thromboembolism associated with peripherally inserted central catheters: a systematic review and meta-analysis. Lancet. 2013;382:311–325.

14. Chopra V. Making MAGIC: how to improve the use of peripherally inserted central catheters. BMJ Qual Saf. 2020;29:879–882.

15. Swaminathan L, Flanders S, Rogers M, et al. Improving PICC use and outcomes in hospitalised patients: an interrupted time series study using MAGIC criteria. BMJ Qual Saf. 2018;27:271–278.

16. Verma AA, Kumachev A, Shah S, et al. Appropriateness of peripherally inserted central catheter use among general medical inpatients: an observational study using routinely collected data. BMJ Qual Saf. 2020;29:905–911.

17. Ullman AJ, Bernstein SJ, Brown E, et al. The Michigan Appropriateness Guide for Intravenous Catheters in Pediatrics: miniMAGIC. Pediatrics. 2020;145:S269–S284.

18. Ray-Barruel G, Cooke M, Chopra V, Mitchell M, Rickard CM. The I-DECIDED clinical decision-making tool for peripheral intravenous catheter assessment and safe removal: a clinimetric evaluation. BMJ Open. 2020;10:e035239.

19. Chopra V, Flanders SA, Saint S, et al. The Michigan Appropriateness Guide for Intravenous Catheters (MAGIC): Results from a Multispecialty Panel Using the RAND/UCLA. Ann Intern Med. 2015;163:S1–S40.

20. Gawande A. The Checklist Manifesto: How to Get Things Right. New York, NY: Holt; 2009.

21. Ray-Barruel G, Cooke M, Mitchell M, Chopra V, Rickard CM. Implementing the I-DECIDED clinical decision-making tool for peripheral intravenous catheter assessment and safe removal: protocol for an interrupted time-series study. BMJ Open. 2018;8:e021290.

22. Popovich KJ, Calfee DP, Patel PK, et al. The Centers for Disease Control and Prevention STRIVE initiative: construction of a national program to reduce health care-associated infections at the local level. Ann Intern Med. 2019;171:S2–S6.

23. Patel PK, Olmsted RN, Hung L, et al. A tiered approach for preventing central line-associated bloodstream infection. Ann Intern Med. 2019;171:S16–S22.

24. Patel PK, Gupta A, Vaughn VM, Mann JD, Ameling JM, Meddings J. Review of strategies to reduce central line-associated bloodstream infection (CLABSI) and catheter-associated urinary tract infection (CAUTI) in adult ICUs. J Hosp Med. 2018;13:105–116.

25. Saint S, Meddings J, Fowler KE, et al. The Guide to Patient Safety for health care-associated infections. Ann Intern Med. 2019;171:S7–S9.

26. Patel PK, Greene MT, Jones K, et al. Quantitative results of a national intervention to prevent central line-associated bloodstream infection: a pre-post observational study. Ann Intern Med. 2019;171:S23–S29.

CHAPTER 5: BUILDING THE TEAM

1. Health care personnel flu vaccination: internet panel survey, United States, November 2012. Centers for Disease Control and Prevention, 2012. Accessed July 24, 2020, at https://www.cdc.gov/flu/fluvaxview/hcp-ips-nov2012.htm
2. Fakih MG, Krein SL, Edson B, Watson SR, Battles JB, Saint S. Engaging health care workers to prevent catheter-associated urinary tract infection and avert patient harm. Am J Infect Control. 2014;42:S223–S229.
3. Farley JE, Doughman D, Jeeva R, Jeffries P, Stanley JM. Department of Health and Human Services releases new immersive simulation experience to improve infection control knowledge and practices among health care workers and students. Am J Infect Control. 2012;40:258–259.
4. Krein SL, Kowalski CP, Harrod M, Forman J, Saint S. Barriers to reducing urinary catheter use: a qualitative assessment of a statewide initiative. JAMA Intern Med. 2013;173:881–886.
5. Greene MT, Fakih MG, Watson SR, Ratz D, Saint S. Reducing inappropriate urinary catheter use in the emergency department: comparing two collaborative structures. Infect Control Hosp Epidemiol. 2018;39:77–84.
6. Saint S, Greene MT, Krein SL, et al. A program to prevent catheter-associated urinary tract infection in acute care. N Engl J Med. 2016;374:2111–2119.
7. Patel PK, Gupta A, Vaughn VM, Mann JD, Ameling JM, Meddings J. Review of strategies to reduce central line-associated bloodstream infection (CLABSI) and catheter-associated urinary tract infection (CAUTI) in adult ICUs. J Hosp Med. 2018;13:105–116.
8. Meddings J, Greene MT, Ratz D, et al. Multistate programme to reduce catheter-associated infections in intensive care units with elevated infection rates. BMJ Qual Saf. 2020;29:418–429.
9. Pronovost PJ, Watson SR, Goeschel CA, Hyzy RC, Berenholtz SM. Sustaining reductions in central line-associated bloodstream infections in Michigan intensive care units: a 10-year analysis. Am J Med Qual. 2016;31:197–202.
10. Ben-David D, Vaturi A, Solter E, et al. The association between implementation of second-tier prevention practices and CLABSI incidence: A national survey. Infect Control Hosp Epidemiol. 2019;40:1094–1099.
11. Dixon-Woods M, Bosk CL, Aveling EL, Goeschel CA, Pronovost PJ. Explaining Michigan: developing an ex post theory of a quality improvement program. Milbank Q. 2011;89:167–205.
12. Meddings J, Skolarus TA, Fowler KE, et al. Michigan Appropriate Perioperative (MAP) criteria for urinary catheter use in common general and orthopaedic surgeries: results obtained using the RAND/UCLA Appropriateness Method. BMJ Qual Saf. 2019;28:56–66.

CHAPTER 6: THE IMPORTANCE OF LEADERSHIP AND FOLLOWERSHIP

1. Collins J. Good to Great and the Social Sectors. New York, NY: HarperBusiness; 2011 (p. 5).
2. Northouse PG. Leadership: Theory and Practice. 8th ed. Thousand Oaks, CA: SAGE; 2018 (p. 5).

3. New findings confirm predictions on physician shortage. Association of American Medical Colleges 2019. Accessed July 24, 2020, at https://www.aamc.org/news-insights/press-releases/new-findings-confirm-predictions-physician-shortage

4. Bennis WG, Nanus B. Leaders: Strategies for Taking Charge. 2nd ed. New York, NY: HarperBusiness; 2007 (p. 20).

5. Saint S, Chopra V. Thirty Rules for Healthcare Leaders. Ann Arbor, MI: Michigan Publishing Services; 2019.

6. Saint S, Kowalski CP, Banaszak-Holl J, Forman J, Damschroder L, Krein SL. The importance of leadership in preventing healthcare-associated infection: results of a multisite qualitative study. Infect Control Hosp Epidemiol. 2010;31:901–907.

7. Mayer JD, Salovey P. What is emotional intelligence? In P. Salovey & D. J. Sluyter (Eds.), Emotional development and emotional intelligence: Educational implications. New York, NY: Basic Books; 1997:3–34.

8. Adams KL, Iseler JI. The relationship of bedside nurses' emotional intelligence with quality of care. J Nurs Care Qual. 2014;29:174–181.

9. Kelley R. In Praise of Followers: Harvard Business Review; 1988. Accessed November 24, 2020, at https://hbr.org/1988/11/in-praise-of-followers.

10. Kelley RE. The Power of Followership. New York, NY: Doubleday Business; 1992.

11. Greene MT, Saint S. Followership characteristics among infection preventionists in US hospitals: results of a national survey. Am J Infect Control. 2016;44:343–345.

12. Van De Waal E, Borgeaud C, Whiten A. Potent social learning and conformity shape a wild primate's foraging decisions. Science. 2013;340:483–485.

13. Rogers EM. Diffusion of Innovations. 5th ed. New York, NY: Free Press; 2003.

CHAPTER 7: COMMON PROBLEMS, REALISTIC SOLUTIONS

1. Pascale R, Sternin J, Sternin M. The Power of Positive Deviance: How Unlikely Innovators Solve the World's Toughest Problems. Boston, MA: Harvard Business Review Press; 2010.

2. Engaging physicians in a shared quality agenda. Institute for Healthcare Improvement, 2007. Accessed July 24, 2020, at https://www.reinertsengroup.com/publications/documents/IHIEngagingPhysiciansWhitePaper2007.pdf

3. Saint S, Kowalski CP, Banaszak-Holl J, Forman J, Damschroder L, Krein SL. How active resisters and organizational constipators affect health care-acquired infection prevention efforts. Jt Comm J Qual Patient Saf. 2009;35:239–246.

4. Saint S, Wiese J, Amory JK, et al. Are physicians aware of which of their patients have indwelling urinary catheters? Am J Med. 2000;109:476–480.

5. Chopra V, Govindan S, Kuhn L, et al. Do clinicians know which of their patients have central venous catheters? A multicenter observational study. Ann Intern Med. 2014;161:562–567.

6. Harrod M, Kowalski CP, Saint S, Forman J, Krein SL. Variations in risk perceptions: a qualitative study of why unnecessary urinary catheter use continues to be problematic. BMC Health Serv Res. 2013;13:151.

7. Grant AM, Hofmann DA. It's not all about me: motivating hand hygiene among health care professionals by focusing on patients. Psychol Sci. 2011;22:1494–1499.

8. Vaughn VM, Saint S, Krein SL, et al. Characteristics of healthcare organisations struggling to improve quality: results from a systematic review of qualitative studies. BMJ Qual Saf. 2019;28:74–84.

9. Clack L, Zingg W, Saint S, et al. Implementing infection prevention practices across European hospitals: an in-depth qualitative assessment. BMJ Qual Saf. 2018;27:771–780.
10. van der Kooi T, Sax H, Pittet D, et al. Prevention of Hospital Infections by Intervention and Training (PROHIBIT): results of a pan-European cluster-randomized multicentre study to reduce central venous catheter-related bloodstream infections. Intensive Care Med. 2018;44:48–60.

CHAPTER 8: JOINING A COLLABORATIVE

1. Michigan Hospital Medicine Safety Consortium (HMS). Accessed July 24, 2020, at https://mi-hms.org/overview
2. Michigan Surgical Quality Collaborative (MSQC). Accessed July 24, 2020, at https://msqc.org/about/
3. Michigan Arthroplasty Registry Collaborative Quality Initiative (MARCQI). Accessed July 24, 2020, at http://marcqi.org
4. Michigan Urological Surgery Improvement Collaborative (MUSIC). Accessed July 24, 2020, at https://musicurology.com
5. Michigan Bariatric Surgery Collaborative (MBSC). Accessed July 24, 2020, at https://www.michiganbsc.org
6. Children's Hospitals' Solutions for Patient Safety (SPS). Accessed July 24, 2020, at https://www.solutionsforpatientsafety.org/about-us/our-goals/
7. Girouard S, Levine G, Goodrich K, et al. Pediatric Prevention Network: a multicenter collaboration to improve health care outcomes. Am J Infect Control. 2001;29:158–161.
8. Haiti's people have strong will to rebuild: CNN;2010. Accessed November 20, 2020 at https://www.cnn.com/2010/OPINION/01/13/danticat.haiti.quake.catastrophe/index.html
9. ØVretveit J, Bate P, Cleary P, et al. Quality collaboratives: lessons from research. Qual Saf Health Care. 2002;11:345–351.
10. Nembhard IM. Learning and improving in quality improvement collaboratives: which collaborative features do participants value most? Health Serv Res. 2009;44:359–378.
11. Schouten LM, Hulscher ME, van Everdingen JJ, Huijsman R, Grol RP. Evidence for the impact of quality improvement collaboratives: systematic review. BMJ. 2008;336:1491–1494.
12. Patel PK, Greene MT, Jones K, et al. Quantitative results of a national intervention to prevent central line-associated bloodstream infection: a pre-post observational study. Ann Intern Med. 2019;171:S23–S29.
13. Meddings J, Manojlovich M, Ameling JM, et al. Quantitative results of a national intervention to prevent hospital-acquired catheter-associated urinary tract infection: a pre-post observational study. Ann Intern Med. 2019;171:S38–S44.
14. Meddings J, Greene MT, Ratz D, et al. Multistate programme to reduce catheter-associated infections in intensive care units with elevated infection rates. BMJ Qual Saf. 2020;29:418–429.

CHAPTER 9: TOWARD SUSTAINABILITY

1. Miller BL, Krein SL, Fowler KE, et al. A multimodal intervention to reduce urinary catheter use and associated infection at a Veterans Affairs Medical Center. Infect Control Hosp Epidemiol. 2013;34:631–633.
2. Pronovost PJ, Watson SR, Goeschel CA, Hyzy RC, Berenholtz SM. Sustaining reductions in central line-associated bloodstream infections in Michigan intensive care units: a 10-year analysis. Am J Med Qual. 2016;31:197–202.
3. Sakihama T, Kayauchi N, Kamiya T, et al. Assessing sustainability of hand hygiene adherence 5 years after a contest-based intervention in 3 Japanese hospitals. Am J Infect Control. 2020;48:77–81.
4. Lieber SR, Mantengoli E, Saint S, et al. The effect of leadership on hand hygiene: assessing hand hygiene adherence prior to patient contact in 2 infectious disease units in Tuscany. Infect Control Hosp Epidemiol. 2014;35:313–316.
5. Petrilli CM, Mantengoli E, Saint S, Fowler KE, Bartoloni A. The effect of merging two infectious disease units on hand hygiene adherence in Italy. J Infect Prev. 2017;18:144–147.

CHAPTER 10: TAKING ON *CLOSTRIDIOIDES DIFFICILE*

1. Finney JMT. Gastro-enterostomy for cicatrizing ulcer of the pylorus. Bull Johns Hopkins Hosp. 1893;4:53–55.
2. Green RH. The association of viral activation with penicillin toxicity in guinea pigs and hamsters. Yale J Biol Med. 1974;47:166–181.
3. Keighley MR, Burdon DW, Arabi Y, et al. Randomised controlled trial of vancomycin for pseudomembranous colitis and postoperative diarrhoea. Br Med J. 1978;2:1667–1669.
4. Bartlett JG. Historical perspectives on studies of *Clostridium difficile* and *C. difficile* infection. Clin Infect Dis. 2008;46(Suppl. 1):S4–S11.
5. Antibiotic resistance threats in the United States. Atlanta, GA: US Department of Health and Human Services, Centers for Disease Control and Prevention; 2019.
6. Dubberke ER, Carling P, Carrico R, et al. Strategies to prevent *Clostridium difficile* infections in acute care hospitals: 2014 update. Infect Control Hosp Epidemiol. 2014;35(Suppl 2):S48–S65.
7. Gut infections are growing more lethal. New York Times. 2012 March 20. Accessed July 24, 2020, at https://www.nytimes.com/2012/03/20/health/gut-infections-are-growing-much-more-lethal.html?searchResultPosition=1
8. Rotjanapan P, Dosa D, Thomas KS. Potentially inappropriate treatment of urinary tract infections in two Rhode Island nursing homes. Arch Intern Med. 2011;171:438–443.
9. Baur D, Gladstone BP, Burkert F, et al. Effect of antibiotic stewardship on the incidence of infection and colonisation with antibiotic-resistant bacteria and *Clostridium difficile* infection: a systematic review and meta-analysis. Lancet Infect Dis. 2017;17:990–1001.
10. Flanders SA, Saint S. Why does antimicrobial overuse in hospitalized patients persist? JAMA Intern Med. 2014;174:661–662.

11. Spellberg B. Antibiotic judo: working gently with prescriber psychology to overcome inappropriate use. JAMA Intern Med. 2014;174:432–433.
12. Rousseau JJ. The Social Contract (Book 1, Section 7). London, England: Penguin; 1762.
13. Edmonds SL, Zapka C, Kasper D, et al. Effectiveness of hand hygiene for removal of *Clostridium difficile* spores from hands. Infect Control Hosp Epidemiol. 2013;34:302–305.
14. Jabbar U, Leischner J, Kasper D, et al. Effectiveness of alcohol-based hand rubs for removal of *Clostridium difficile* spores from hands. Infect Control Hosp Epidemiol. 2010;31:565–570.
15. Oughton MT, Loo VG, Dendukuri N, Fenn S, Libman MD. Hand hygiene with soap and water is superior to alcohol rub and antiseptic wipes for removal of *Clostridium difficile*. Infect Control Hosp Epidemiol. 2009;30:939–944.
16. McDonald LC, Gerding DN, Johnson S, et al. Clinical practice guidelines for *Clostridium difficile* infection in adults and children: 2017 update by the Infectious Diseases Society of America (IDSA) and Society for Healthcare Epidemiology of America (SHEA). Clin Infect Dis. 2018;66:987–994.
17. DeFilipp Z, Bloom PP, Torres Soto M, et al. Drug-resistant *E. coli* bacteremia transmitted by fecal microbiota transplant. N Engl J Med. 2019;381:2043–2050.
18. Wilcox MH, Gerding DN, Poxton IR, et al. Bezlotoxumab for prevention of recurrent *Clostridium difficile* infection. N Engl J Med. 2017;376:305–317.
19. Rohde JM, Jones K, Padron N, Olmsted RN, Chopra V, Dubberke ER. A tiered approach for preventing *Clostridioides difficile* infection. Ann Intern Med. 2019;171:S45–S51.
20. Dubberke ER, Rohde JM, Saint S, et al. Quantitative results of a national intervention to prevent *Clostridioides difficile* infection: a pre-post observational study. Ann Intern Med. 2019;171:S52–S58.

CHAPTER 11: THE FUTURE OF INFECTION PREVENTION

1. Saint S, Meddings J, Fowler KE, et al. The guide to patient safety for health care-associated infections. Ann Intern Med. 2019;171:S7–S9.
2. Patel PK, Gupta A, Vaughn VM, Mann JD, Ameling JM, Meddings J. Review of strategies to reduce central line-associated bloodstream infection (CLABSI) and catheter-associated urinary tract infection (CAUTI) in adult ICUs. J Hosp Med. 2018;13:105–116.
3. Patel PK, Olmsted RN, Hung L, et al. A tiered approach for preventing central line-associated bloodstream infection. Ann Intern Med. 2019;171:S16–S22.
4. O'Grady NP, Alexander M, Burns LA, et al. Summary of recommendations: guidelines for the prevention of intravascular catheter-related infections. Clin Infect Dis. 2011;52:1087–1099.
5. Beattie M, Taylor J. Silver alloy vs. uncoated urinary catheters: a systematic review of the literature. J Clin Nurs. 2011;20:2098–2108.
6. Saint S, Elmore JG, Sullivan SD, Emerson SS, Koepsell TD. The efficacy of silver alloy-coated urinary catheters in preventing urinary tract infection: a meta-analysis. Am J Med. 1998;105:236–241.

7. Pickard R, Lam T, MacLennan G, et al. Antimicrobial catheters for reduction of symptomatic urinary tract infection in adults requiring short-term catheterisation in hospital: a multicentre randomised controlled trial. Lancet. 2012;380:1927–1935.

8. Sager R, Kutz A, Mueller B, Schuetz P. Procalcitonin-guided diagnosis and antibiotic stewardship revisited. BMC Med. 2017;15:15.

9. Meddings J, Saint S, Krein SL, et al. Systematic review of interventions to reduce urinary tract infection in nursing home residents. J Hosp Med. 2017;12:356–368.

10. Trautner BW, Grigoryan L, Petersen NJ, et al. Effectiveness of an antimicrobial stewardship approach for urinary catheter-associated asymptomatic bacteriuria. JAMA Intern Med. 2015;175:1120–1127.

11. Mody L, Greene MT, Meddings J, et al. A national implementation project to prevent catheter-associated urinary tract infection in nursing home residents. JAMA Intern Med. 2017;177:1154–1162.

12. DeCherrie LV, Wajnberg A, Soones T, et al. Hospital at home-plus: a platform of facility-based care. J Am Geriatr Soc. 2019;67:596–602.

13. Federman AD, Soones T, DeCherrie LV, Leff B, Siu AL. Association of a bundled hospital-at-home and 30-day postacute transitional care program with clinical outcomes and patient experiences. JAMA Intern Med. 2018;178:1033–1040.

14. McCain J. Hospital at home saves 19% in real-world study. Manag Care. 2012;21(11):22–26.

15. Saint S, Trautner BW, Fowler KE, et al. A multicenter study of patient-reported infectious and noninfectious complications associated with indwelling urethral catheters. JAMA Intern Med. 2018;178:1078–1085.

16. Leuck AM, Wright D, Ellingson L, Kraemer L, Kuskowski MA, Johnson JR. Complications of Foley catheters—is infection the greatest risk? J Urol. 2012;187:1662–1666.

17. Kashefi C, Messer K, Barden R, Sexton C, Parsons JK. Incidence and prevention of iatrogenic urethral injuries. J Urol. 2008;179:2254–2258.

18. Lee T, Yang H, Haneuer DA, Wan J. Preventing traumatic urinary catheter insertion through a computerized ordering system: quasi-experimental study from a tertiary academic center. Hosp Pract Res. 2018;3:28–31.

19. Bearman G, Bryant K, Leekha S, et al. Healthcare personnel attire in non-operating-room settings. Infect Control Hosp Epidemiol. 2014;35:107–121.

20. Petrilli CM, Mack M, Petrilli JJ, Hickner A, Saint S, Chopra V. Understanding the role of physician attire on patient perceptions: a systematic review of the literature—targeting attire to improve likelihood of rapport (TAILOR) investigators. BMJ Open. 2015;5:e006578.

21. Landry M, Dornelles AC, Hayek G, Deichmann RE. Patient preferences for doctor attire: the white coat's place in the medical profession. Ochsner J. 2013;13:334–342.

22. Jennings JD, Ciaravino SG, Ramsey FV, Haydel C. Physicians' attire influences patients' perceptions in the urban outpatient orthopaedic surgery setting. Clin Orthop Relat Res. 2016;474:1908–1918.

23. Andersen MJ, Flores-Mireles AL. Urinary catheter coating modifications: the race against catheter-associated infections. Coatings 2019;10(1):23.

24. Noyce JO, Michels H, Keevil CW. Potential use of copper surfaces to reduce survival of epidemic methicillin-resistant *Staphylococcus aureus* in the healthcare environment. J Hosp Infect. 2006;63:289–297.

25. Rai S, Hirsch BE, Attaway HH, et al. Evaluation of the antimicrobial properties of copper surfaces in an outpatient infectious disease practice. Infect Control Hosp Epidemiol. 2012;33:200–201.

26. Implementing filtering facepiece respirator (FFR) reuse, including reuse after decontamination, when there are known shortages of N95 respirators. Centers for Disease Control and Prevention. Accessed August 10, 2020, at https://www.cdc.gov/coronavirus/2019-ncov/hcp/ppe-strategy/decontamination-reuse-respirators.html

27. Zoutman D, Shannon M, Mandel A. Effectiveness of a novel ozone-based system for the rapid high-level disinfection of health care spaces and surfaces. Am J Infect Control. 2011;39:873–879.

28. Ameling J, Greene MT, Quinn M, Meddings J. Pilot testing a bedside patient safety display to increase provider awareness of the "hidden hazards" of catheters and wounds. Infect Control Hosp Epidemiol. 2020;41(1):s351–s352.

29. *Candida auris*. Centers for Disease Control and Prevention 2019. Accessed July 24, 2020, at https://www.cdc.gov/fungal/candida-auris/index.html

30. Global monoclonal antibody therapeutics market will reach USD 218.97 billion by 2023. Zion Market Research. Accessed July 24, 2020, at https://www.globenewswire.com/news-release/2018/04/10/1467446/0/en/Global-Monoclonal-Antibody-Therapeutics-Market-Will-Reach-USD-218-97-Billion-by-2023-Zion-Market-Research.html

31. Varrone JJ, Li D, Daiss JL, Schwarz EM. Anti-glucosaminidase monoclonal antibodies as a passive immunization for methicillin-resistant *Staphylococcus aureus* (MRSA) orthopaedic infections. Bonekey Osteovision. 2011;8:187–194.

32. Mitsuma SF, Mansour MK, Dekker JP, et al. Promising new assays and technologies for the diagnosis and management of infectious diseases. Clin Infect Dis. 2013;56:996–1002.

33. The Fat Drug. New York Times. 2014 March 9. Accessed July 24, 2020, at https://www.nytimes.com/2014/03/09/opinion/sunday/the-fat-drug.html

34. McGuckin M, Waterman R, Storr IJ, et al. Evaluation of a patient-empowering hand hygiene programme in the UK. J Hosp Infect. 2001;48:222–227.

35. Montoya A, Schildhouse R, Goyal A, et al. How often are health care personnel hands colonized with multidrug-resistant organisms? A systematic review and meta-analysis. Am J Infect Control. 2019;47:693–703.

36. Patel PK, Mantey J, Mody L. Patient hand colonization with MDROs is associated with environmental contamination in post-acute care. Infect Control Hosp Epidemiol. 2017;38:1110–1113.

37. Cao J, Min L, Lansing B, Foxman B, Mody L. Multidrug-resistant organisms on patients' hands: a missed opportunity. JAMA Intern Med. 2016;176:705–706.

38. Shanafelt TD, Boone S, Tan L, et al. Burnout and satisfaction with work-life balance among US physicians relative to the general US population. Arch Intern Med. 2012;172:1377–1385.

39. Beach MC, Roter D, Korthuis PT, et al. A multicenter study of physician mindfulness and health care quality. Ann Fam Med. 2013;11:421–428.
40. Fortney L, Luchterhand C, Zakletskaia L, Zgierska A, Rakel D. Abbreviated mindfulness intervention for job satisfaction, quality of life, and compassion in primary care clinicians: a pilot study. Ann Fam Med. 2013;11:412–420.
41. Gilmartin H, Goyal A, Hamati MC, Mann J, Saint S, Chopra V. Brief Mindfulness Practices for Healthcare Providers-A Systematic Literature Review. Am J Med. 2017;130:1219 e1–e17.
42. Kiyoshi-Teo H, Krein SL, Saint S. Applying mindful evidence-based practice at the bedside: using catheter-associated urinary tract infection as a model. Infect Control Hosp Epidemiol. 2013;34:1099–1101.
43. Gilmartin H, Saint S, Rogers M, et al. Pilot randomised controlled trial to improve hand hygiene through mindful moments. BMJ Qual Saf. 2018;27:799–806.
44. IBM's Watson is better at diagnosing cancer than human doctors. Wired. 2013, February 11. Accessed July 24, 2020, at https://www.wired.co.uk/article/ibm-watson-medical-doctor

APPENDIX A: ANN ARBOR CRITERIA FOR URINARY CATHETERS IN HOSPITALIZED MEDICAL PATIENTS

1. Meddings J, Saint S, Fowler KE, et al. The Ann Arbor Criteria for Appropriate Urinary Catheter Use in Hospitalized Medical Patients: Results Obtained by Using the RAND/ UCLA Appropriateness Method. Ann Intern Med. 2015;162:S1– S34.

APPENDIX B: MICHIGAN APPROPRIATE PERIOPERATIVE (MAP) CRITERIA FOR URINARY CATHETER USE

1. Meddings J, Skolarus TA, Fowler KE, et al. Michigan Appropriate Perioperative (MAP) criteria for urinary catheter use in common general and orthopaedic surgeries: results obtained using the RAND/UCLA Appropriateness Method. BMJ Qual Saf. 2019;28:56–66.

APPENDIX C: TWO-TIERED APPROACH TO PRIORITIZE INTERVENTIONS FOR CATHETER-ASSOCIATED URINARY TRACT INFECTION (CAUTI), CENTRAL LINE–ASSOCIATED BLOODSTREAM INFECTION (CLABSI), AND CLOSTRIDIOIDES DIFFICILE INFECTION (CDI)

1. Meddings J, Manojlovich M, Fowler KE, et al. A tiered approach for preventing catheter-associated urinary tract infection. Ann Intern Med. 2019;171:S30–S37.
2. The Targeted Assessment for Prevention (TAP) Strategy. Centers for Disease Control and Prevention. Accessed February 11, 2021, at https://www.cdc.gov/hai/prevent/tap.html

3. Saint S, Meddings J, Fowler KE, et al. The Guide to Patient Safety for health care-associated infections. Ann Intern Med. 2019;171:S7–S9.

4. Patel PK, Olmsted RN, Hung L, et al. A tiered approach for preventing central line-associated bloodstream infection. Ann Intern Med. 2019;171:S16–S22.

5. Rohde JM, Jones K, Padron N, Olmsted RN, Chopra V, Dubberke ER. A Tiered Approach for Preventing *Clostridioides difficile* Infection. Ann Intern Med 2019;171:S45–S51.

APPENDIX D: GUIDE FOR PATIENT SAFETY (GPS) TOOLS FOR CAUTI, CLABSI, AND CDI

1. Saint S, Meddings J, Fowler KE, et al. The Guide to Patient Safety for health care-associated infections. Ann Intern Med. 2019;171:S7–S9.

2. Saint S, Gaies E, Fowler KE, Harrod M, Krein SL. Introducing a catheter-associated urinary tract infection (CAUTI) prevention Guide to Patient Safety (GPS). Am J Infect Control. 2014;42:548–550.

3. Fletcher KE, Tyszka JT, Harrod M, Fowler KE, Saint S, Krein SL. Qualitative validation of the CAUTI Guide to Patient Safety assessment tool. Am J Infect Control. 2016;44:1102–1109.

4. Catheter-associated urinary tract infection (CAUTI) Guide to Patient Safety (GPS). CatheterOut. Accessed August 25, 2020, at https://www.catheterout.org/cauti-gps.html

5. Central line-associated bloodstream infection (CLABSI) Guide to Patient Safety (GPS). ImprovePICC. Accessed August 25, 2020, at https://www.improvepicc.com/gpsclabsi.html

6. *Clostridioides difficile* infection (CDI) Guide to Patient Safety (GPS). PSEP. Accessed August 25, 2020, at https://psep.med.umich.edu/gpscdi.html

APPENDIX E: MICHIGAN APPROPRIATENESS GUIDE FOR INTRAVENOUS CATHETERS (MAGIC) CRITERIA

1. Chopra V, Flanders SA, Saint S, et al. The Michigan Appropriateness Guide for Intravenous Catheters (MAGIC): Results from a Multispecialty Panel Using the RAND/UCLA. Ann Intern Med. 2015;163:S1–S40.

Page numbers followed by *b, f,* or *t* indicate boxes, figures, or tables, respectively.